LIVING WITH DEMENTIA

Chronicle Herald Readers' Responses

"Darce Fardy gives us the special gift of sharing his Alzheimer's journey. His insights and observations offer a unique perspective. If we have the eyes to see and ears to hear Darce, we can celebrate his gift to us of insights that offer us the potential to be the game changers in these global health challenges. Thanks are not enough from us to Darce Fardy as he shares his journey." — **H. H.**

"I am always inspired and reassured after reading Darce Fardy's columns on living with dementia. Thank you, Darce, for your tenacity in continuing to share insights and facts while living your unique journey. Bravo to all your networks of family, friends, professionals, and even strangers for supporting and encouraging you to be living your life fully. Let's not be embarrassed, as Darce says. Rather, let's share our unique journeys and celebrate life, while living." — **S. B.**

"Thank you for carrying Darce Fardy's accounts of aging with Alzheimer's over the years. It meant a lot to readers who are dealing with aging friends suffering from this horrid disease. He told of a deeply personal journey that touched your readers' hearts." — **P. M.**

"Hooray for Darce Fardy. ...Mr. Fardy's chronicle of living with dementia is a must-read. He is a courageous individual and a talented writer. With so many families being touched by this daunting condition, his continuing account of daily challenges, hopes, and desires is a revelation. The support he needs and receives from family and friends is key to his quality of life. The pragmatism and humour displayed in his anecdotes and his willingness to share the difficult bits is a unique contribution to our understanding of the process. We owe him our gratitude for truthfully sharing the journey." — **M. H.**

"In one column, Darce Fardy pretty much covered the curriculum of an Alzheimer's course! Perhaps, most important, is the positive self-attitude Darce reflects in his writing. His sense of humour, I truly hope, will serve him and his family for time to come." — **S. B.**

"Having lost a cherished loved one to this most heinous and debilitating of diseases, I'm well aware of the toll it takes on both the one afflicted and their family.

I commend Mr. Fardy in his approach to dealing with dementia, which he has done with poignancy, humour, and courage. As a journalist, he is a credit to his craft; as a person, an inspiration to humanity." —**D. J.**

LIVING WITH DEMENTIA

The Collected Columns of
DARCE FARDY

Foreword by Kenneth Rockwood, MD

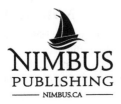

NIMBUS
PUBLISHING
— NIMBUS.CA —

Nimbus Publishing Limited
3660 Strawberry Hill St
Halifax, NS, B3K 5A9, (902) 455-4286, nimbus.ca

Nimbus Publishing is based in Kjipuktuk, Mi'kma'ki, the traditional territory of the Mi'kmaq People.

Printed and bound in Canada
NB 1737

These columns first appeared in the *Halifax Chronicle Herald* between 2014 and 2020; they are reprinted here with permission.
All images courtesy Peter Fardy.

Editor: Angela Mombourquette
Cover design: John van der Woude, JVDW Designs
Interior design: Rudi Tusek

Library and Archives Canada Cataloguing in Publication

Title: Living with dementia : the collected columns of Darce Fardy / by Darce Fardy ;
    foreword by Kenneth Rockwood, MD.
Other titles: Collected columns of Darce Fardy
Names: Fardy, Darce, author.
Identifiers: Canadiana (print) 20240421515 | Canadiana (ebook) 20240421531 |
    ISBN 9781774713365 (softcover) | ISBN 9781774713372 (EPUB)
Subjects: LCSH: Fardy, Darce. | LCSH: Dementia—Patients—Nova Scotia—Biography.
    | LCGFT: Autobiographies.
Classification: LCC RC521 .F37 2024 | DDC 616.8/3110092—dc23

IN SUPPORT OF

Société **Alzheimer** *Society*

NOVA SCOTIA

All net proceeds from the sale of this book will be donated to the Alzheimer Society of Nova Scotia.

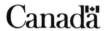 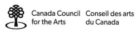 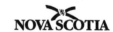

Nimbus Publishing acknowledges the financial support for its publishing activities from the Government of Canada, the Canada Council for the Arts, and from the Province of Nova Scotia. We are pleased to work in partnership with the Province of Nova Scotia to develop and promote our creative industries for the benefit of all Nova Scotians.

Contents

2017

Darce Fardy: A Life in Photos

2018

Foreword

It is an honour to write this foreword. I am delighted to have had the chance to read through all of Darce's columns. (I make a point of always addressing patients formally, but from the get-go, Darce would have none of that—"Mr. Fardy is my father.") His columns bring pleasure, not rarely leavened with poignancy. Darce's voice remains clear throughout, even as, over the eight years of writing, we can see subtle changes. Still, we always get some sense of the man behind the words. We can see how essential parts of him persisted, notably his good humour, his equanimity, his great respect for people, and his deep love for his wife and family. Even for a Newfoundlander—even for "one of we"—Darce was a natural storyteller. His understatement, apt turn of phrase, his distillation of life lessons into objects as unlikely as an onion, are the hallmarks of a person who can spin a yarn.

In training here in Halifax to become a geriatrician, I had the great privilege to work with the late Dr. John Gray, who in the early 1980s founded the Division of Geriatric Medicine at Dalhousie University and its first clinical outpost at what then was known as Camp Hill Hospital. The essence of the person with the diagnosis was an important theme in his teaching. Doctor Gray always framed the disclosure of what a dementia diagnosis means in a particular way. Having told the patient that their symptoms most likely were explained by their having Alzheimer's disease—remember, this was before there was any type of medical treatment—he would make this point:

"You are the same person you were just now before I told you this diagnosis. You care about the same things you have always cared about. It has taken a long time for you to develop this problem, and it will likely take a long time for it to get worse. Take this to heart. What is important to you now can sometimes change, but the people whom you love, you will always love. And the people who love you now will always love you. This disease does not change the essence of who you are."

Being able to see the essence of the person is a great gift. Despite Dr. Gray's example, I know it is not one that I was always able to employ. With Darce though, it was easy. Through some combination of his wife, Dorothea, family, friends, genes, grace, luck, mobility, neighbours, privilege, and treatment, he was a "star" patient. Darce was able to comport himself well and act on his own terms more than most, even unto the end.

His work made a contribution, and so can this book. It makes it clear that dementia is not the end, and that a good quality of life can remain possible for a long time. Reading this will make clear that when we see a person living with dementia, we must aim to see the person, not just the dementia.

Given his understanding that not everyone with dementia was as fortunate as he, Darce took on advocacy. His career—first as a journalist, and later as Nova Scotia's Freedom of Information Officer—equipped him well for the work.

As you will see, he put that experience to great use. For a few years after he no longer needed to come to the memory clinic ("You're too good for me," I'd told him) if we met up it was typically at a conference or other public gathering where he was a featured speaker. As with this book, Darce was brave. He shared his struggle with the public. He admitted that even though he was doing well, he still recognized any number of small losses. That such losses were made harder by how buses were scheduled, crosswalk lights positioned, or public spaces designed motivated him to point to how, as individuals, as a province, and as a society, we can do better. I ran into Darce one time after I'd returned from a course on architecture and design for dementia. He was well ahead in thinking about accessibility, well aware that when we made spaces better for people living with dementia—easier to navigate and maintain, more likely to nudge people to come together or to pause on a busy day—we were making those spaces better for everyone.

The progression of Darce's dementia also makes clear what sorts of medical treatments we need to improve the lives of people living with dementia. Even now, a lot of emphasis is placed on memory, and especially on new learning. This is not wrong—consistent improvement in memory would be a great blessing. Darce's story, however, tells us that this is somewhat misguided. Even when his memory was not good, for the most part his social comportment—his good graces, and some insight—saved him. In the trade, this goes by the name "executive function." Executive function is measured mostly indirectly, by accounts of whether someone has initiative or can newly be rude, is uncharacteristically irritable, is able to plan, or has insight. Even less directly, it is measured by so-called "frontal lobe tests." These are at some remove from those characteristic habits, looks, movements, interests, and irritants that make us recognizably who we are. When I listen for accounts of treatment to judge whether what we are prescribing is "working" I listen for short phrases that can mean so much: "My [mother/father/wife/husband/brother/sister] is back"; "They are more like their old self"; "They are the person I always knew." The many lessons for us from this include that we need treatments, environments, and social interactions that can make being "more like their old self" a routine expectation, not the less common and more remarkable event that it is now.

In that way, as in many others, the experience of Darce Fardy is a lesson for us all. Don't believe me though: find out for yourself. And as you read the columns, be sure to keep an eye out for the onions.

Kenneth Rockwood, MD

Professor of Geriatric Medicine and Neurology
at Dalhousie University and Senior Medical Director
of the Frailty and Elder Care Network at
Nova Scotia Health

Introduction

In 2013 my father was diagnosed with dementia. He was eighty-one years old and was by all appearances in fine health for a man his age. Nonetheless, neither he nor we (his family) were surprised by the diagnosis. His memory had clearly been in some early stage of decline.

Over the following years, there was nothing sudden or dramatic about what we observed. But over time he had an increasing tendency to repeat himself or ask questions to which he knew (or should have known) the answers. As an example, he would sometimes ask me or my sisters if we had ever met someone who had in fact been a lifelong family friend. The diagnosis just made it official.

Dad was never much of a hand-wringer, so not only did he accept the situation and the likely consequences; he practically embraced them. He had read somewhere that people with dementia presented too great a risk for other drivers, their passengers, and pedestrians. He voluntarily gave up his car keys before anyone asked him to. He never complained about the resulting lack of independence and, since he had always been an avid walker, he kept on with that.

This is not to say he was not worried. He had seen the toll the disease had taken on two of his siblings, but he never allowed any sense of inevitability to govern how he would approach each day.

As a former journalist, it was a natural act for him to decide to document his experience from that point forward. He pitched the idea to one of the editors at the *Halifax Chronicle Herald*, and over the next six years almost seventy of his columns were published.

As his family, we were all quite keen on this writing project because it gave him such purpose. He was always preoccupied with what he would write about next and seemed to always have at least one column "in the can."

Perhaps what surprised him (and us) the most was how much attention the columns attracted. We heard from countless friends, acquaintances, and strangers about how much they appreciated reading them. Wherever he went, people would recognize him, introduce themselves, and thank him for what he was doing. They would also often share their own personal stories. Dad loved these encounters and would often write about them.

What this revealed, perhaps more than anything else, was the extent to which dementia touched other people's lives. Everyone seemed to have a story about a loved one who was dealing with it. While every one of these stories was unique, people found comfort in reading about someone else's journey. The positive, yet unplanned, benefit of the columns was that they helped destigmatize the disease and bring discussion of it out in the open.

I was frankly a little taken aback by all the accolades, especially since he so often seemed to simply write about "what happened last weekend," with hardly a mention of dementia. Reading them again—this time in sequence and as a consolidated set—has revealed a greater relevance than I first saw. I now have a better understanding of why they meant so much to so many.

Our family had always been very open about things, so this was a welcome realization. As the disease and its symptoms slowly progressed, nothing changed in this regard. Dad retained his sense of humour and the self- deprecation that accompanied it. Jokes about his condition were far from taboo and were, in fact, encouraged. He was always a voracious reader, and that drew my mother to observe that he would now only need two books: he could read one and then, by the time he finished the second, the first one would be new to him again!

Humour and a positive attitude may have helped keep the worst symptoms at bay for a while, but we all knew the disease could not be defeated. Sure enough, every passing year saw Dad's mental and physical conditions decline. We learned that those two things come hand-in-hand and, following a number of falls and related injuries, his increasing fragility became the more pressing concern.

Despite these physical challenges, my father kept writing his columns, which serve as a window on his deteriorating condition. In the following pages, you may notice this in the quality and coherence of his writing. He kept it up as long as he could, with an increasing amount of editorial support from my mother. By early 2020 his ability to piece together a coherent five hundred–word essay was out of reach. He died two years later.

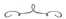

In early 2014, just after his diagnosis, my father completed a project he had been working on for several years. It was the story of his life, intended not as a formal autobiography for a wider audience, but rather as a record of his life for his six grandchildren, all of whom were at the time too young and preoccupied to naturally express much interest in the topic. He told us he wished he'd known about his own grandparents but had no written record to which he could refer, so he wrote his story down so it would be there when his family wanted it. For the fun of it, we self-published it so he could present it to each of the grandkids in a more "professional" format.

Perhaps prophetically, this was his final entry in that story:

> That last paragraph was written only weeks before I was diagnosed with dementia—early dementia. Family was the first to notice. I put it down to the fact that I was a poor listener. My GP got me an appointment with our memory clinic. Dorothea came along, of course, but so did Peter and Donna (Sheila was in Toronto). Our Toronto friends Bob and Christine Culbert have a daughter Alison, a GP. When I told her about the dementia, she said she sees many of her older patients and asked if I would keep a progress diary for her to use in

her practice. I said I would, and I have now started. And I provide them to family as well.

So, there we are! Doctor Rockwood, the head of the memory clinic observed that at eighty-one closing in on eighty-two it's likely that "something else will get me first," before I and my family have to deal with serious symptoms of dementia.

This book picks up the story from there.

My father would take great joy in knowing that other families take comfort from his writings. I hope you will see why the columns and this book are titled *Living with Dementia*—not dying from it.

Peter Fardy

2014

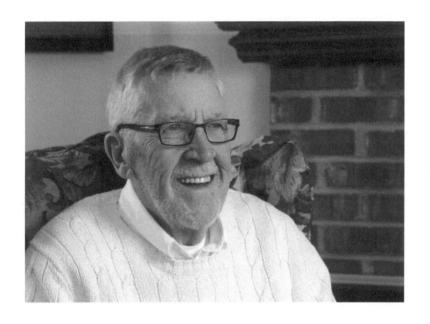

1

Darce's Diagnosis

Published February 21, 2014

Darce Fardy has always been a storyteller. He worked as a journalist with the CBC for forty years. After that, he made sure other journalists were able to uncover the truth, too, in his role as the province's freedom of information officer. Now Fardy is telling his own story about his decline into dementia. The is the first in a series of articles about his journey.

I worked until I was seventy-five, then founded the non-profit group promoting open government for which I was awarded a Queen's Jubilee Medal in 2012. I stepped down at eighty-one. I was diagnosed with dementia before I reached eighty-two.

I am told that before I start telling my dementia story I should talk about my past experiences. I'm told it helps the reader.

I was born in the east end of St. John's, NL, seventeen years before Newfoundland reluctantly agreed to let Canada join us. We lived in the shadow of the Catholic basilica and our street was named for a former archbishop. We had a family of eight, including my parents, in a very small house. An aunt also lived with us. In that town at that time people did not discuss their health and, in fact, hid their illnesses. It was nobody's business.

My business was journalism. I was with the CBC for forty years in four provinces. All of those years I was a news reporter and supervisor before moving into journalism management at the network level. (That may explain why I volunteered to do this column without being asked. I thought it was a good story.)

When I retired, I was offered the opportunity to become Nova Scotia's first freedom of information review officer. For a journalist this was like striking gold. I was to receive applications from people asking me to review government decisions made in response to their requests for information. It was a contract position carrying a daily rate which remained the same throughout my six years in the job...$150 per day worked. No vacation pay. Not even a weather day. I think I submitted my bill every week. This was all fine with me. I had a CBC pension, and I loved the job.

I think I was good at it as well, which explains what appeared to be efforts to make me quit. I probably would have taken the job for lunch money. I walked away when I concluded the Justice Department was playing with me.

Back to dementia.

My family began to notice that I seemed to be having trouble remembering names, directions, and the like. I put this down to the fact I was a poor listener. That's true, but there was more. My wonderful GP, Frank Lo, sent me off to the local memory clinic. Like any curious person, I wanted to know what went on at the clinic and I wanted to share the experience with all the family living in Halifax—not just my wife, who would be attending anyway.

I must say in all modesty the decision to invite everyone was brilliant. It seems odd to say so, but it was a good experience for all of us. The family discussed with staff what was happening while I was going from room to room for tests.

I was first taken away and asked to answer a list of questions. I thought the first question unfair: What's today and what's the date? My "examiner" laughed when I complained that thousands of people would have stalled on that one. But I soldiered on.

She told me my wife was answering the same questionnaire, but I never did get to see my wife's answers. I mention this only to point out how relaxed and friendly the whole process is. I know I failed miserably the walk across the room in my stocking feet. Other clinic staff were called in as witnesses. (I challenge readers to try walking corner-to-corner in their living rooms with their shoes off and not wander off the track.)

The tests took about three hours. When it was over, the head of the clinic, Dr. Kenneth Rockwood, a wonderful man, spent more than an hour with the whole family, answering questions from all of us. A young doctor friend of mine in Toronto told me that some of her patients were reluctant to take the tests.

She was one of those who encouraged me to go public with this story.

I start with an advantage. Walking and exercise and reading newspapers and books help slow down brain deterioration. My wife and I read the *Chronicle Herald* and the *Globe and Mail* every morning. Fortunately, there is no Sunday paper, because both weekend papers take two days to read. We also pick up *Metro*.

I'm just finishing Paul Wells's fine book on the politics of Stephen Harper and his crew. I got five or six books for Christmas. I used to belong to a gym and will return. I also enjoy walking and have walked more than half an hour every morning for years. (Best to do it in the mornings before other stuff comes up.)

A visit to a physiotherapist is part of the process. I got detailed instructions from a wonderful woman on what exercises I should do. I now have weights for daily exercises and a stationary bike to use in cruddy weather...the kind we have had since November.

I grew up the youngest of four brothers and two sisters. I am the only one of the boys left. The other three died younger than I am, all with cancer. One of them, a brilliant guy who was a professor at Memorial University of Newfoundland's medical school, had advanced dementia as well. Only the oldest sibling, a sister, is still alive after a severe stroke and is in a nursing home. I am often the only visitor she recognizes.

The other day I couldn't remember the name of a street I often walk down. It's a major get-out-of-town street. One of my family used to live on a side street. I walked it the other day but deliberately avoided looking at the street name. I still haven't brought it up.

I want to thank my family for their support.

I was pleased when I learned that my grandchildren know about their granddad's health problems. Grandson Seamus, seeing an advantage he couldn't resist, challenged me to a memory game he found online. He beat me handily and so did his nana.

I'm gearing up for another round.

2

Fostering the Dementia Debate

by Kenneth Rockwood, MD

Rockwood is a geriatrician at Nova Scotia Health (formerly Capital Health)
and an Alzheimer scientist at Dalhousie University in Halifax.

Published February 21, 2014

D arce Fardy is doing something brave. He is talking about being diagnosed with Alzheimer's disease, which is the most common cause of dementia. Fardy is not just drawing attention to this problem. He is giving us a new way to think about it. He is challenging us in how to live well with dementia.

His timing is impeccable. The new provincial government aims to develop a dementia strategy in just one year. This is ambitious. There is no shortage of tough subjects. On some, the public is engaged. We know that many people with mild dementia can drive, but no one with moderate dementia can.

As the [drivinganddementia.ca] website shows, we must plan in every case that, at some point, driving will stop. In long-term care, we know that the wait-list policy encourages people to go into nursing homes sooner than they really need to. Combining that with institutional incentives to select people with the fewest impairments means that often it is easiest to get care when you don't really need it. [A reminder: this was originally written in 2014–Ed.]

Overcoming those perverse incentives will take work, but the high rates of institutional care in Nova Scotia oblige us to not just build more beds.

Perverse incentives also abound in private assisted living, a parallel system of long-term care. There, people pay premium dollars "in case something happens." But when it does, they must pay extra for an expensive service menu. Some facilities transfer patients to hospital on the smallest pretense, and then refuse readmission on the grounds of their being "too heavy to care for." No mention is made that a lot of their money is now gone.

So Nova Scotians use our most expensive resource—acute-care hospital beds—to backstop predatory practices. This must change.

Other key topics get little airing. Some physicians opt out of knowing anything about dementia, claiming that the drugs don't work. (The evidence is that they do for many, but not for all, and that trying them is usually the only way to know.) Many other physicians have become fully engaged in dementia care. At present, they do so out of professionalism, not profit: dementia care is strikingly underpaid.

When dementia goes unrecognized and untreated, routine hospital care is much less effective. We miss the chance to treat people who are likely only to be confused for a short period while they are sick with other problems. Not recognizing dementia can even make some expensive care harmful. Patients undergo "routine" procedures at higher risks than they realize. That is because preoperative assessments of risk now mostly focus on the heart and lungs, not the brain. And we need to define successful treatment in not just technical terms. Success is defined by whether people live better afterward.

And when people choose not to have expensive procedures, we need to offer them other forms of care. We shouldn't just expect them to, like the patient in the Stephen Leacock essay, "quietly die, or quietly get better," but either way to not bother us.

Fardy wants us to tackle all this, but rightly he wants us to get beyond it. The new dementia strategy must also focus on living well with dementia. It's not just that better care for people with dementia will oblige practices that make care better for everyone. We need to think about how we design our public spaces.

Even though exercise is essential to prevent and treat dementia, in many public buildings stairs are hard to find and not attractive to use. Making our communities more walkable for people with dementia makes them more walkable and easier to navigate for everyone. Likewise for making homes and apartments easier to grow old in. If we can make it normal to ask people who look lost whether they need help, that helps everyone.

Fardy wants us all to understand the need for listening with care and for seeking out and enjoying some quiet time. He is telling us that living well with dementia requires paying attention to what matters. This is just as true at the policy level as it is at the personal. He is doing us a great service. We should avail of it.

3

The Silences are Deafening

Published March 22, 2014

My wife and I were at our friends' house recently, and on the kitchen counter were some cocktail napkins bearing a mock motto that read: "The positive side to memory loss: you meet new people every day."

For my wife and me, it said everything.

It reaffirmed our decision to make public my diagnosis of dementia, and we knew then that the couple we were visiting were real friends—they got it!

The *Chronicle Herald* asked me earlier this year if I would consider writing a series of columns tracing my progress since being diagnosed. I'm happy to do so and this is my second crack at it. My first column attracted attention across the country and below the border. The local CBC television and radio networks were also interested in my decision to "go public," and after my first column was published, on one of my regular walks on Quinpool Road, several people approached me after reading about or hearing about my diagnosis.

My barber admonished me to come to him for a styling before my next photograph is taken. The woman who runs the nearby gas station told me about her father's condition. A woman I know called me to say how much she appreciated our decision to go public. She cared for a husband with dementia for many years. He was diagnosed long before he was my age. I'm eighty-one.

I am a regular visitor to the Halifax Seaport Farmers' Market every Saturday. I usually go alone, but now that I don't drive, my wife, Dorothea, took me a few weeks ago and decided to come in with me. We expected to attract some attention. Some approached us and others, unfortunately, may have been uncertain about what to do. I understand that people may be uncomfortable, but I hope they get over it. I'm sure they wouldn't be uncomfortable approaching a person diagnosed with cancer. One seller at the market, seeing my wife, observed that she probably needs to come with me now.

She doesn't and likely won't.

On the matter of driving, I have decided to stop cold turkey for two reasons: I may be distracted (perhaps more than the minds of the drivers texting), and I expect if there were an accident my insurance company would be loath to honour my policy.

Naturally, we are quite interested in if or how friends and acquaintances approach me. Though I have heard from dozens of friends and former associates both here in Nova Scotia and across the country and from the United States, I have not heard from some I was associated with over recent years here in Halifax. I don't know why that is. I'm not offended by this but, rather, just wonder why. Perhaps some of them are uncomfortable as well. If so, that's too bad. All of the reaction I got—by email, phone, or in person—was positive.

My wife, a better observer of my performance than I am, says she has noticed no decline in the past few months. I appear to have no problems remembering names of people I knew years ago. But recently, I received an email from someone I knew at the CBC when I worked there twenty years ago. I had seen her since both of us retired, so I remember her well. But when I was telling my wife that I had heard from her, I couldn't immediately come up with her name.

There are other minor lapses; one that I haven't fessed up to. I make hot cereal every winter morning. It requires cereal and water only to prepare it. Then into the microwave. Quite simple. So one morning, I reached for the little measuring cups I have been using for years. One is larger than the other by a little. And then I froze.

Which one was for the water and which for the cereal? Then it struck me: Dorothea wrote out instructions for preparing certain meals and stuck them to the back of the cupboard doors years ago. And there was the one for my cereal, just two lines—the small cup was for the cereal and the larger one for the water. It was posted years ago and the ink was fading.

All in all, there has been no deterioration in the past few months.

When the CBC Radio program *The Current* called me, they sensibly asked my wife to join in the interview. I have said many times that when dementia happens, the family is affected as much as the person diagnosed. Dorothea does not share the same enthusiasm for public attention that her husband, a former journalist, does. But she recognizes that people need to hear her story as well as mine. We have both accepted an invitation to appear at an international conference being held in Halifax in June. An organization called the Elder Mediation International Network is hosting the Seventh World Summit and Symposium on Mediation with Age Related Issues.

My wife and I have dedicated much of our time to slowing down the progress of this disease. I have rejoined my gym after a four-year hiatus. Slim Gyms doesn't need my endorsement, but they know of my "condition" and have tailored my exercises to fit my needs.

In my first column I noted that I couldn't remember the name of a street, one of the busy get-out-of-town streets. I noted one of the family used to live on a side street. I also told you I refused to look at the street name on my walks. Well, wouldn't you know it?

I unintentionally looked. Jubilee Road.

Also in my first column, I had mentioned that we had included our grandchildren in the discussion about my dementia. The guy who challenged me to a memory game and beat me badly somehow made a point of listening to his nana and granddad on *The Current* in the classroom. A granddaughter wrote a presentation on Alzheimer's for her class project.

My youngest grandchild wondered if his granddad would remember his name, and his mother consoled him.

4

Daily Exercise is the Best Medicine

by Dr. Kenneth Rockwood

Published March 22, 2014

Darce Fardy continues his public service in describing his journey with Alzheimer's. As one of his doctors, there's little I can say specifically about him beyond that. Even with his being public, every patient can expect their physicians to maintain confidentiality.

Even so, Darce's article today raises three questions: What do memory symptoms mean? Why does the approach to treatment put so much emphasis on exercise? What can we say to people who now have dementia?

At the memory clinic, I always tell young doctors that memory complaints are only important to the patient: the symptoms don't help us make a diagnosis. Many people with dementia believe that their memory is fine. The research on "subjective memory complaint" tells us that vastly more people have memory complaints than will develop dementia. So if someone notices memory problems and this prompts them to take steps to prevent dementia, that's good. But if all they do is worry about their memory, that is not helpful.

It's easy to encourage people to prevent dementia. Much of what seems to work amounts to living well. This means doing most things in moderation. Except smoking: no smoking. Being socially engaged is important. So, too, is living a mentally stimulating life. Reading the newspaper every day is good, as is regular contact with friends.

Going out—to social groups, church groups, or live theatre—appears to be better than watching television. For the really ambitious, challenges like learning a second language or taking up a musical instrument appear to offer protection. Even so, as good as those are, physical exercise is best.

The optimal amount of exercise for effective prevention seems to be about forty-five minutes a day, five days a week. Three of those days should include twenty to thirty minutes of weightlifting or other resistance training like push-ups.

If you are starting from nothing, this sounds like a lot. But the whole point is to start. Any regular exercise is better than none. Get out and walk. And walk with someone: most people exercise more when another person is with them. If Nova Scotia is to adopt a dementia strategy, programs that encourage people of all ages—but especially over age fifty—to get out and get active will be a good place to start. So, too, will training programs for people to build up their exercise capacity gradually. The first three months are key. After that, it becomes a habit—even an enjoyable one.

Exercise is not just for prevention. It is also a mainstay of treatment. We often suggest a physiotherapy assessment first. Many people have a condition or injury that can limit certain types of exercise. The physiotherapy assessment lets them find out which exercises they can do safely. It's a way to ensure that no one is too old or too inactive to exercise. What they need is a program that works for them.

In exercise as treatment, having a coach is key. "It's coaching, not nagging" is what I tell patients. And a playing coach is best: someone who does the exercise program alongside the person with dementia. This can be an excellent way for a friend to help.

Many people want to help, but they don't know what to say. Some people are so afraid of dementia that they become afraid of people with dementia—even people they've known all their lives. Darce is showing us that, especially at the early stages, and especially for people who respond to treatment, there's not a lot to be afraid of.

But it's still scary. There's no formula for how to start the conversation. The best advice is to just start. Make the call, or go see them, or even just don't look away when they see you. Go up, talk to them. Pick up on the cues. Don't be afraid to introduce yourself if they don't seem to know you. "It's good to see you" is often better than "How are you?"

Sometimes people are all talked-out about dementia. Ask about something else or share a story. Don't be afraid to give a compliment. If you feel there is some way you can help, make the offer. Be specific: "Can I pick you up to go to the mall/church/game?" is often better than: "Let me know if there is something I can do." Think how much better off we are for Darce actually doing what he's doing.

Let's follow his lead.

5

I Am Neither Victim nor Hero

Published May 24, 2014

I recently had coffee with a learned and younger friend in a café on Quinpool Road. We both spotted a guy we knew walking past the window. I remembered his name; my friend couldn't. This provoked so much laughing we attracted the attention of other customers.

And that's the way it should be.

It doesn't mean he has dementia, and it doesn't mean I don't. That being said, it will be difficult for me to resist reminding him of that episode when next we meet.

Some time later I was having a coffee with a friend when other good friends came into the café. I confess I did wonder for a moment if I could handle the situation and remember all three names. I did, but if I hadn't, I know that I would have been rescued quickly and graciously by either party.

I am discovering that remembering names may be my most challenging issue at this time. There's no question it can be embarrassing but, there you go, it is what it is. It doesn't happen with family or friends I see regularly. It usually happens when someone I know well pops out of the past.

Recently, I went to a fundraiser with my son and daughter-in-law to support the wonderful Churchill Academy in Dartmouth. It was my first "public function" since I revealed my dementia and I never gave it a second thought until, when I arrived, it occurred to me that people might be giving me a second look, and some might be feeling a little uncomfortable. In fact, more than a few people approached to say hello—some I knew and others I didn't. I imagine my son was asked how I was doing by some others, but I wasn't embarrassed, and they weren't embarrassed.

There is no reason for those with dementia to avoid people, and that's the message I am trying to get out. I haven't had an uncomfortable moment with people since I went public. In fact, I have received countless emails of encouragement. One of them, which I received recently, was from a woman I had never met but whose father worked with me at the CBC. She wrote:

> I want to thank you and Dorothea for your transparency as you both face a future that includes Alzheimer's. I read your two articles in the *Chronicle Herald* and hope there are more to come. I can't help but think that your experiences and willingness to share them serve to help and inspire others.
>
> I was struck by the fact that many people have used the words "brave" and "courageous" to describe the fact that you and Dorothea have gone public with your story. Given the stigma associated with Alzheimer's, it seems fitting that people view your efforts through the lens of courage, but I hope we'll see a day when talking about Alzheimer's is no braver than discussing heart disease. It's the stigma that silences both people with Alzheimer's and their families.

I hope I've made it clear that I don't see myself as a victim or a hero.

We have lots of support from family and beyond and socialize regularly with wonderful friends. Our close family friends have dropped in from Toronto in two shifts to see for themselves how we're doing, and more are coming.

Since I started my story, thanks to [the *Chronicle Herald*] and other media, I have met with the Alzheimer Society of Nova Scotia and will be attending a summertime conference. We were both interviewed for an online Alzheimer's group. And we have been invited to speak to an international conference being held later this year in Halifax. My wife and I are both willing to be helpful where we can.

Dorothea and I and the family have now started the discussion relating to what to do now: sell the house and rent a one-floor apartment or make changes to our home to accommodate what ails me. Some argue that we should stay where we are and where we've been for twenty-some years. With all of our moving about, this is the first house we have really settled into. We've never stayed this long in one home since we were married. On the other hand, it's a three-storey home—lower floor, first floor, and second floor, not including an attic. We'll see what happens.

I have mentioned before that we have kept our grandchildren involved. We did not want them overhearing hushed conversations about their granddad. Their nana and I get no sad looks from them because we have taken the time to take them into our confidence.

My eldest, Gabrielle, who lives in Toronto, contacted me recently to tell me that, in her psychology class, students were asked to do a presentation on someone who inspires them and why. She chose her granddad, got a 95 percent on the paper, and whimsically concluded I must have inspired her high mark as well.

6

Should We Stay
or Should We Move?

Published July 5, 2014

As I predicted in my last column, Dorothea and I have begun wrestling with the inevitable question: do we stay where we are or move into a one-level apartment?

The personal advantage of moving to an apartment is obvious—no clearing snow or spreading salt on an icy driveway and steps, no putting out the garbage, no more maintenance issues, no stairs to navigate. Our home has three flights of stairs: from the lower level to the main level, to the bedroom level, and to the attic. Washer and dryer, bathroom, and a sewing room that doubles as a bedroom on the lower level: kitchen, living room, den, dining room, and front and back porches on the ground floor; and three bedrooms and a bathroom on the top level. The stairs to the attic are found in the smallest room, which is used as an office but can double as a bedroom.

Anyone would conclude that this presents a bit of a challenge for any couple, let alone one that includes a woman in her mid-seventies and a man in his early eighties with dementia (I reached eighty-two since my last column).

We set about looking at a number of apartments and concluded we wanted one in an area where we knew we would enjoy living: near the waterfront, within walking distance of a supermarket, the farmers' markets, and the wonderful boardwalk. We found the apartment we wanted with a wonderful panoramic view of the harbour and a large kitchen that Dorothea, who likes to entertain family and friends, would not be comfortable without. The apartment would not be available for a few months, but we were all right with that.

So we began preparations. We talked to real estate people and began preparing our home to be sold. We gave away surplus furniture, cleared out our closets and the attic, and took clothes and appliances to the Salvation Army in three or four carloads. A few hundred books went to a used bookstore. The owner said he would try to sell some and give the rest to a nearby Salvation Army store that would give them away to anyone who wanted one.

We've discovered that clearing a house for sale is a Herculean task. And now it's done.

We had a plan in case the house sold before an apartment was available. We would stay through the week at our son and daughter-in-law's cottage on weekdays and, when they went to the cottage, we would move into their home. (They may be hearing this here for the first time!)

As you may understand, this was a fairly emotional time. We had lived in this home longer than we had lived in any other over our fifty-five years together. Dorothea had wallpapered the halls, bedrooms, and bathrooms after we moved in, which was certainly a huge investment. A skilled friend built wonderful mantels and made new steps to the basement. But, we concluded, moving was inevitable.

And then I awoke one morning and considered that we lived close to our son and daughter-in-law and two of our grandchildren (across the street, in fact) and within a ten-minute walk of one of our daughters and two more of our grandchildren. As one would expect, they dropped in regularly. That would not happen if we moved into an apartment on the waterfront. I know Dorothea had this in mind, as did I, but we felt the decision to move was a good and necessary one.

And then we changed our minds over morning coffee.

I got up first that morning and put to paper the new scenario and proposed some questions: Did it make sense to put ourselves in a situation where there would be no unplanned drop-ins? Would we see our family as often? Would Dorothea, the quintessential nana, be comfortable being out of reach? It became a rather emotional coffee break.

While we were wrestling with the new scenario, we came home one day to find a note from our daughter-in-law, Carol. She had crossed the street to get an onion and left us a note to confess. I figured she would be unlikely to head to the waterfront for an onion. I suppose if we had to protect our onions, we could change the password on our home security system! (That seemed a bit extreme. Besides, Carol is an experienced nurse with a wonderful reputation; a good person to have as a neighbour.)

On a more practical level, a lot of other planning accompanied our change of heart. The future might dictate the necessity of moving the laundry to the top floor and putting a toilet room in our back porch. We believe that can be done.

And so we have decided to stay in our home...and leave the onions at risk.

7

Darce and Dorothea Offer Lessons for Living

by Kenneth Rockwood, MD

Published July 5, 2014

D arce Fardy and his wife, Dorothea, are putting their onions at risk in order to live well. Darce addresses the issue of where to live—and with it, of how to live. They have opted to stay put in familiar surroundings.

Doing so means living with some risk. What if things get worse and one of them needs a wheelchair? Or help around the house? Or can't navigate the stairs in their multi-level home?

They are not in denial. They are adapting their home. They are getting the laundry and bathroom facilities organized for single-level living, and they are doing this before they need to. They are acting on a plan, not reacting to events that might threaten to over-take them.

They are decluttering; getting rid of what is no longer needed is not just a physical act, it is an emotional act, too. Moving out extra furniture, packing up hundreds of books, and clearing out clothes can feel like giving up, but they are showing us that these chores are also a sign of taking stock. They are looking forward and finding a new focus. Some readers, who understand the need for taking stock all too well, will envy them: at least they can plan together.

Darce and Dorothea have decided to mitigate some of the risks of staying put. They reckon it will be worth it to have the benefit of familiarity and of close contact with friends and neighbours—even at the risk of having onions borrowed while they are out.

Not everyone facing this decision will decide to stay put.

As we continue to build homes that are not age-friendly, many people will surrender independence as the way to reduce risk. They will move because they see no other option. But options exist and many more will come. Population aging will drive innovations in technology, materials, structure, and design. Age-friendly design is in its infancy. Enclosing steps to the outdoors, for example, makes perfect sense in our climate, but how often is something this simple done? The growing demand for age-friendly building, and the low supply, make it ripe for the sort of innovation imagined by the Ivany report [*The Report of the Nova Scotia Commission on Building Our New Economy*, February 2014].

Age-friendly innovation will work not just for older adults, but for everyone, and so it will come. The question is whether Nova Scotia will get in now or wait until it is all worked out somewhere else. Unless we see opportunity in the huge demands that dementia is making worldwide, we will not prosper. In fact, right now, I'm worried that we will not even cope.

Although I saw Darce initially to make a diagnosis and suggest a treatment plan, I am not following him in my clinic. These days, I only see him when we're speaking at public meetings. That's because he is the sort of patient to whom I say: "You're too good for me." Instead, my geriatrician colleagues and I focus on people who have not yet been diagnosed, or whose problems are more complicated than average.

Things will get a lot busier.

The G7 has focussed on dementia, which has led to more initiatives around the world—some even trickling down to Nova Scotia. Now, thankfully, the province is developing a dementia strategy which is expected in less than a year. (See Afterword for a current follow-up on these points.)

There is a lot of work to be done in the meantime. One piece of work is to train more specialists in geriatric medicine. Incredibly though, right now, the plan for next year is to have no new training posts. The plan, once again, is to turn away Nova Scotia physicians who want to complete their training in internal medicine and geriatric medicine here.

No one actually denies what is coming. Everyone understands how long the training takes. But unlike Darce and Dorothea, the thinking seems to be that we can wait. Wait until there is a new policy, wait for the latest reforms, or wait until events overtake us.

Let's learn from Darce and Dorothea about how to size up risk, plan ahead, and act. If we all just keep waiting, a lot more than a few onions will be at risk.

8

Get Thee to the Gym

Published September 13, 2014

I'd like to spend a little time paying homage to the humble walking cane.

With family "encouragement," I have recently been using a cane. (I used one some ten years ago after I had a hip replacement but haven't needed it in years). I am told that dementia can at times cause some unsteadiness when walking, so I've taken my cane, more often than not, every day for some months now. And that raises new issues. Dorothea reminds me to take it but isn't there to remind me to bring it home. My average is not great. Up to now, I have left the cane in supermarkets, hardware stores, restaurants—you name it.

If I've been to only one locale, it's pretty easy to trace. But recently I had been in five when I noticed it missing—took two days before I found the thing. Dorothea bet I wouldn't find it. She was wrong! Though she was prepared to write off the cane, she agreed to drive me to try another stop. Moments later, I returned to the car, triumphantly holding the damn thing over my head.

Sometimes I'm lucky. In Toronto recently, I left my cane in a store on Bloor Street. I had walked from my daughter's home to get the morning papers. As I sashayed up the sidewalk, I heard a shout behind me. A customer saw the abandoned cane and chased me with it. (Who says Torontonians are unfriendly!)

Most recently I forgot to take it with me when I was getting off a bus. A passenger alerted me and hurried to the exit to pass it over like an Olympic torch. The driver scowled.

I now have three canes and a shillelagh. But using an alternate to go pick up the missing one presents its own peculiar problem—walking home with two. Recognizing how much I enjoy urban walking, summer and winter, I have a spiked cane for winter and, believe it or not—because I really like walking outdoors—I have spikes on a pair of my shoes, if needed. However, with one hand occupied by a cane, my capacity for carrying stuff is limited, so I wear a backpack. At times like this, decked out for walking, cane in hand, I look more like Edmund Hillary than Fred Astaire.

Unsteadiness is also a focus of exercises I do to help slow the advance of dementia. When I was diagnosed by the memory clinic, I was dispatched to a physiotherapist who outlined the exercises I should do to deal with my problems. This list was delivered to the gym I attend. The physio plan I use is called the Cognitive Impairment Exercise Program. It says research has concluded that "physical activity [is] beneficial in all stages of dementia" and should include "a combination of endurance, strength and balance."

Lack of balance, of course, is easier to spot than the other two.

The program requires that my exercise be balanced too—aerobic, strength, and flexibility, as well as balance. Aerobics includes brisk walking, treadmill, stationary bicycle, cycling, and swimming. These are exercises I can do without help from the gym staff. I have a stationary bike and weights at home. We are told that this activity doesn't need to be "intense." A person should be able to talk throughout. Strength training, on the other hand, should require effort to complete. Fortunately, it advises there should be NO PAIN—in bold capital letters. I found that comforting. Although I can practise balance anywhere any time, the program assures me, the staff of my gym have found ways to help in that area.

The document ends with a Summary of a Successful Program: Exercise with someone else in a comfortable setting, do a half-hour of cardio and a half-hour of resistance, balance, and flexibility, and change things periodically. And that's what I'm doing.

At my gym, there are twenty stations, and most of them involve the exercises I have been advised to do. Among them, under the welcome watch of gym staff, are a leg press, a chest press, and an exercise that strengthens arms. The balance board, mockingly called the wobble board, can be a bit of a challenge. My overseer stands by in case I go ass over kettle (that hasn't happened, thank heavens) and consoles me that I am improving. And I tend to agree with him. A "ladder" stretched across the floor also improves balance as I jump on and off at every rail. Other stations are designed to improve the lower back as well as arm and leg strength and improve hip and knee flexibility.

So that's what I'm doing, and I believe the advice of the physiotherapist to be sound.

Going to a gym may be difficult for some at the start. Soon you realize the room is full of sweating and grunting individuals just like you. Lots of seniors around. I hope all readers will take the advice of the clinic that regular, organized exercise will either allay or delay dementia. "Get thee to a gym" is good advice for everyone!

Meanwhile, my awkward relationship with the cane will continue. Despite my intemperate remarks, there'll be no "cane" mutiny.

9

Exercise is a Cornerstone of Dementia Prevention

by Kenneth Rockwood, MD

September 13, 2014

Darce Fardy's adventures in Alzheimer's disease continue. As always, his experience is instructive. He again reminds us of the benefits of going to the gym. This cannot be emphasized too strongly. Physical exercise is the cornerstone of treatment, and of prevention. Hopefully, a clear role for exercise will be recognized in the province's much-anticipated dementia strategy. It might even not be too late for the architects designing the many new buildings going up in Halifax. To start, perhaps they can be encouraged not to hide the stairs but to make it natural to take them.

Darce describes ways to overcome the awkwardness that many people might feel in taking up an exercise program for the first time in decades. He is right: it is usually very easy to fit in with all the other sweating seniors. Most are too busy working through their own programs to use any energy to mock. He also reminds us that exercise is not just about going to the gym; it involves being active outside. That activity should not stop during the winter—another important note for architects, developers, and planners and whoever else needs to be persuaded not to make obstacles of our sidewalks.

Most interesting to me are his comments about first using a cane and then so often losing it. Scientists now recognize that how people move can be affected with Alzheimer's disease. In fact, changes in mobility and balance can occur early in the course of the illness. Previously, we recognized that in advanced dementia, people walk slowly, with short steps and a narrow base. Now we understand that, even before dementia is evident, some have difficulty walking and talking at the same time. Others have problems in maintaining their balance, especially when getting in and out of chairs or bed. For many people—and not just those with dementia—a cane can have a dramatic impact, not just on how a person walks but on their confidence in walking.

Losing the cane is another matter. Why would a dementia expert find this interesting? It seems so simple. People with Alzheimer's disease have memory problems. When they lose their cane, isn't it just a matter that they forgot where they put it? What could be so interesting about that?

Talking to people who witness someone misplacing commonly used and needed objects every day makes it easy to see how complicated a problem this can be. To start, it's less about forgetting where something was put. More often, the issue is remembering the need to pick it up again at the time that it is put down. This is a useful distinction, because here memory merges with other things the brain does.

Our brains plan and make judgments and pay attention. Misplacing objects is probably better understood as an aspect of this, rather than as an aspect of memory itself. Such functions use a different mix of brain chemicals than memory does. Understanding which ones are in play can help us better understand how dementia unfolds, and how we might treat it.

In this light, I read Darce telling us that "moments later, I returned to the car, triumphantly holding the damn thing over my head" as being especially important. It provides a clue about what happens in the brain when objects are misplaced.

Let me emphasize that point. There is still fundamental work to be done in understanding Alzheimer's disease by listening carefully to people who have it and to the people who care for them. Their stories can then be set against how we understand brain function, using careful tests and new technology such as the IWK's magneto-encephalography (MEG) machine, which measures the magnetic fields produced by the brain's electrical currents. Hopefully, the province's new dementia strategy will seek to support research for which existing Nova Scotia resources are particularly well suited. This is just one of many examples.

Many readers are likely to have shuddered at the description of the lost cane. That is because misplacing objects is common not just with Alzheimer's disease; it happens to many people as they get older. (Or even before they get older; I know one colleague who, for at least the last twenty years, has given thanks daily for the stereotype of the absent-minded professor. Without that, he might have long since been institutionalized.)

Losing a cane is not the same as losing a mind. Many of dementia's symptoms merge into everyday experience. This can frighten off some people who otherwise might be able to reach out and help. The trick is to put the anxiety to good use. For most people, it should mean talking to their doctor about how to best protect their brain.

Start with listening to Darce Fardy and taking up an exercise program.

10

Fine, Thank You.
And Your Name Is?

Published November 1, 2014

S o how am I doing? That's a question I'm sure my family hears
every day. So I'll try to tell you.

But first, permit me a digression.

I recently met a woman. Jean Fraser, a long-time friend of our
friends, lives in New Glasgow, NS, where we met her recently. At
ninety-three, she lives alone in her lovely traditional home that features lace curtains, doilies on the furniture, and, in an adjoining
room, a computer. When she effortlessly got out of a plush chair to
join us for fish and chips, I asked about a cane. She said she doesn't
have one but is very careful. I almost fell out with her over that.

When she was told about my columns, she asked my friend to
be sure to send her "the link." This wonderful woman has eleven
years on me, and she keeps a watchful eye on a 106-year-old lady in
a nearby nursing home. She's an inspiration.

So how am I doing more than ten months after my diagnosis? I
assume that means I have had dementia for a year or longer, and
honest self-examination can be difficult. As they say about lawyers
representing themselves in court, they have a fool for a client. When
I'm asked how I'm doing, I always say "fine." But I'm told that's been
my stock answer, even after I woke from hip replacement surgery
some years ago. I have to admit it can be bloody frustrating to forget
the names of people I know well, but I'm not sure this is noticed yet.

It's happening more often lately. I suspect good friends are helping me without flagging it. Recently, I temporarily lost the name of a friend I had just had a coffee with. Invariably, friends tell me that this has happened to them from time to time. It probably has, but I know this is different. Dorothea certainly has noticed some deterioration. I fear I may have to keep my phone numbers and security codes in my wallet.

Recently, I was asked the family name of my daughter in-law, Carol. I went blank and showed it. I could see this caused some discomfort to the person who had asked me. I came up with the name just as he was moving on and shouted the answer to him. I'm sure those who heard the holler wondered what I was on about.

Of course, I don't want people hesitating to ask me such questions. It's probably good therapy. My mother used to say there was "too much commotion" in our house when her six children, all fifteen months apart, were together in a small house. I have found that commotion can cause me some discomfort. Not enough, of course, to discourage family gatherings. And perhaps "commotion" is not the word, because when the grandkids are around I usually cause most of it.

Speaking of commotion, our wonderful farmers' market on the Halifax waterfront is the place to find it, and I go there as often as I can. I take the bus to get there. I don't drive anymore, and I am disinclined to use Dorothea as my constant driver.

It's becoming a bit of a challenge since I began using a cane. It leaves me with just one hand for everything else—getting on the bus, slipping the ticket in the box, and shopping around at the market. But with the help of my knapsack, I can do it all.

Just to be perverse, I buy a coffee and find a place to sit, looking out on the harbour. It must look like part of a *Seinfeld* episode to those who notice. And they do. At one counter, I asked the bemused proprietor to hold my cane while I picked up some bread. As it happens, she is no stranger to dementia in her family.

I guess when I'm unable to put my thoughts on paper I can conclude my condition is worsening. That's not happening yet, and

I'm grateful to the *Chronicle Herald* for its encouragement. I enjoy writing. I guess it's good therapy. I try to approach my travails with good humour, and my wife and I have many wonderful days with great friends. But I know—and they likely know—that down the road things may be a lot more difficult for my family.

I am fortunate to have a family doctor the memory clinic describes as someone who knows the dementia file well. Dorothea and I went to see Doctor Frank recently to discuss some fallout from the one particular pill I take. It was unfriendly to me. (As expected, Dorothea comes on these visits with me.) He decided to give me a prescription for a second pill, and I haven't used it long enough to learn its effects. But I was left to understand that I could no longer take alcohol. I didn't take much, at least in later years, but I like an occasional beer.

So at Thanksgiving dinner, I joined the grandkids having a Coke or a chocolate milk. I'm tempted to appeal to Doctor Ken, the expert, for a dispensation, but I won't, and I won't cheat.

11

Strength in the Power of Two

Published December 27, 2014

It's inevitable, I suppose, that I should wonder, twelve months after I was diagnosed with dementia, whether I am becoming too needy and self-centred. Fortunately, Dorothea is a very practical woman and would rein me in if required. I usually go with her on errands, even shopping sometimes. And I go with her when she picks up our grandchildren. But why not? That's not to say we don't do things on our own. But we do a lot more together than we ever did since we were married.

Not much in the way of transgressions since my latest column, though I did put ice cream in the fridge instead of the freezer. It's a venial transgression. Perhaps a sign but not of much consequence. I suppose there will be other lapses.

As you know, the memory clinic and my family doctor, Frank, have provided me with advice to stay active and I do so at the gym and by walking. But I think I have found another way that must be helpful. I have mentioned in earlier columns about the time Dorothea and I now have for reading. Every morning, Dorothea and I read the *Chronicle Herald* and the *Globe and Mail* and chat about stories that would be of interest to both of us. We are regular listeners to and viewers of what we call "current affairs programs"— *The Current* and *The Sunday Edition* on CBC Radio, *The Fifth Estate* on CBC-TV, and the suppertime newscasts. And we subscribe to

Maclean's and *The Walrus* and other newsy magazines. We check our iPad, of course, but for us there is no substitute for picking up a newspaper or newsmagazine. And we always have a book in progress. I am now reading Chantal Hebert's new book on the Quebec referendum. If I can plow through Quebec politics, I should be able to handle anything. All of that information take-in has to be good for the brain cells.

Dorothea and I both worked outside the home for a long time. I was seventy-five when I could stay home, but even then I spent another five years working with a non-profit coalition promoting open government. I travelled a lot while with the CBC. On two occasions I was away from home for an entire year. No wonder I don't know how to run a house! Dorothea had retired earlier (from outside the home, not inside, I hasten to add). So we enjoy the new time we have.

The highlight for both of us since my last column appeared was a provincial conference on a dementia strategy organized by the Alzheimer Society here in Halifax. I was invited to speak. Some two hundred people, a large majority of them women, attended the conference. Dorothea and I were sought out by many during the conference, and we were impressed and touched by the devotion these people had to improving the lives of those with dementia. We squeezed into a table for lunch and heard one of the women tell us how much she loved the four or five women that she cared for in a "home." She said she loved them as she would her grandparents. She missed them on her days off. I feel she represents the passion of most of those attending.

My contribution to the conference was a public chat with a young woman, aptly named Sara Jewell, who had moved into her parents' house for six years while her family faced the dementia of her father. Another young woman, Dawn, a busy young RCMP officer with a family, spoke to the conference. She also cares for her mother, who has dementia and lives with the family. She mentioned it because it was an integral part of her talk, not because she was looking for plaudits.

People were particularly interested in meeting Dorothea. They had met her only through my columns. I introduced her in an unorthodox way. The stage I was to mount before speaking had steps but no rail. A herculean challenge for me. Fortunately, we spotted this earlier. So Dorothea stood to help me up to the stage. We laughed. It was not an awkward moment. I introduced her to the meeting as I stood securely on the stage and before she took her seat. I think she has forgiven me for that. As might be expected, she had many questions to ask some of the experts at our table—power of attorney, banking, and other issues that will arise as my dementia progresses. On the question of forgetting passwords and security numbers—or worse, losing credit cards—a doctor at our table suggested to her that, when it comes time, I could wear a medical alert bracelet with the necessary access numbers engraved on the inside. On other important issues, she will seek the advice of a lawyer who was sitting at our table during the conference.

With the editor's indulgence, again, I'd like to tell the story of another remarkable person we've met in the past twelve months. Linda and her husband's children have long left their beautiful old home in Northport, a Cumberland County, NS, community where my son, daughter-in-law, and their family have a cottage. Linda is still available, of course, to help with the grandchildren. She decided a while ago that she would write the history of her community. She had never attempted a book before. The years to 1940 are now complete and she has started researching the remaining years. She's learned that many people, including cottagers, are looking forward to the next edition.

Linda is one of those many people who take it upon themselves to adopt a leadership role in their community. When the new Northport bridge was completed last summer, she knew who it should be named for, and she set out to make sure that happened. Larry Brander, who had Down syndrome, died a while ago. Everyone in town knew him. He used to wander around town and drop into people's kitchens, uninvited perhaps, but welcome. As a clergyman once said at the funeral of a Down syndrome brother of my friend, "he knit the community together." And in Northport, they always knew where Larry was; now they and others will remember him as they cross his bridge. On a personal note, my younger sister Mary, with Down syndrome, wandered around the neighbourhood in St. John's, NL, seventy years ago, picking flowers from people's carefully manicured gardens. Everyone knew her and there were never any complaints. As for Linda, anyone who can prevail over a bureaucracy for good reasons is to be commended. Some notables may have hoped to have the bridge named for [themselves], but Linda prevailed.

Meanwhile, I came away from the Alzheimer's conference convinced that if I have to move to a home, Dorothea will feel secure that she can travel from time to time to visit relatives and friends in St. John's and Toronto. The rest of our family will also be at ease. I will be in good hands.

Soon Dorothea and I will be getting legal advice on how best to prepare for the advance of my dementia...stuff on wills, banking, and the like. It's fortunate I am able to go with her, though she is much more familiar with wills and the like than I am.

I hope to have an opportunity to tell you about it in another column.

2015

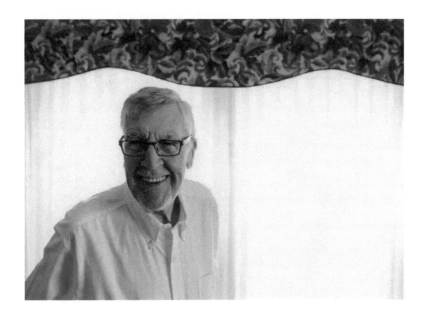

12
Plans and Feelings Can Co-exist

Published February 7, 2015

And so it goes, as more plans are made for what is likely to happen as my dementia advances. This is the practical stuff. In my last column, I told you that we would be going to see a lawyer who was familiar with dementia issues. And we did. We wanted to discuss what measures we needed to take for a time when my dementia has progressed to a point where I am unable to make decisions for myself. We all recognized that I am some distance from that point but being too early was better than being too late.

We both had met this lawyer when she spoke at an Alzheimer's conference we attended. Although we had prepared living wills when I was seventy-five, those documents needed to be looked at again with our future in mind. I was, of course, participating in this meeting. I can say emphatically that I have no problems exercising the changes we will likely have to make. I expect that when the time comes, I will be a co-operative guy.

We had already decided we would offer our bodies to a medical school. Our lawyer pointed out that the medical school would likely want to examine the brain of someone with dementia, particularly when that person had kept a public diary of sorts. I think my columns have provided much of that information. I would like to put myself in a position where I could help in pursuit of a cure for dementia. I know it sounds ghoulish, even perhaps a bit self-serving, but that's the kind of conversation we need to have before the inevitable. It's important for everyone, but, in my case, it's important to have those conversations now.

Our next stop was the bank, where we discussed with our banker how we might deal with the possibility that I lose my wallet or reach a point where I might make inappropriate withdrawals or purchases, using either my debit or credit cards. It seems the answer is to limit the daily maximum I can access on my debit card, and to lower my credit card limit. This decision has the added advantage of protecting us should someone else attempt to use either card. Our accounts have now been flagged by the bank so that any attempt to exceed these amounts using my card will be brought to the bank's attention. I was able to reassure my family that I had no difficulty accepting these pecuniary restraints.

Over Christmas, we sat down with our son and two daughters and went over our new wills and our own wishes should we become incapacitated. They have now read everything, and we have answered all their questions. I found all of this very satisfying, and I believe the family did as well.

It was a first for all of us. It was salutary. All of this may seem surreal, but this is no *cris de coeur*. I'm still enjoying life and talking too much. I don't think I am any crankier than I ever was.

So far, the family is doing well relating to a husband, father, and granddad whose memory is fading. We had all six grandchildren—ages ten to eighteen—and their parents with us at Christmastime. And on Boxing Day we were able to invite close friends to come and meet the whole family. At that reception, Gabrielle, our eldest grandchild, chose to migrate during the evening between the adults in the living room and her five cousins in the den, all of them with their heads down, exercising their thumbs on iPhones and watching *The Big Bang Theory*.

Gabrielle, who lives in Toronto and attends university in Washington, DC, on a soccer scholarship, now drives, just as her granddad has stopped driving. Grandson Seamus, who lives near us, has his driver's licence too. For Christmas, he received the keys to our car with a note attached reading, "Granddad's chauffeur." *Tempus fugit*!

The only awkward moment over the holidays was when I was dumb enough to wonder aloud about next Christmas. I should have predicted the reaction. Oh well! Even Granddad's not perfect.

I have now been through two Christmases and fifteen months since I was diagnosed, with not much new to report. (I will need a dispensation if I repeat stuff I have mentioned in other columns.) I sometimes forget names. I try to bluff my way through it. Good friends are willing to help me out in such a subtle fashion that I don't even notice the interjection.

Although I can find my way to any part of the city, I frequently do not remember street names. There's no cause to fret over that yet. I walk to and from the gym, even in –15°C temperatures. When the sidewalks look iffy, I arm myself with a spiked walking cane. So, with a sharp stick and a muffler masking part of my face, I probably look threatening to kids going off to school.

Now for the "fools walk in where angels fear to tread" bit. As you can imagine in the situation Dorothea and I are in, patience is required of both parties. Dorothea, of course, needs more patience than the "patient," but the patient requires some too. (Here I enter the "angels fear to tread" arena.) After driving in Halifax for many years (I quit only a year ago), I "knew" the best routes to take downtown and the best places to park. Not surprisingly perhaps, Dorothea finds different routes to take and has different favourite parking spots. And she doesn't appear to need a co-pilot. Well, believe or not, I have managed to stay out of it.

It's tough sometimes, though.

A final story, again at my peril. In my era, most men I knew never did the wash, except occasionally for the dishes. So I delicately pointed out to Dorothea the other day that I was running short of clean unmentionables. She assured me that there's a cache of clean underwear, pajamas, etc., available for unexpected travel or emergency. I should have known.

As time goes by, I guess it's natural for me to think more about how all this will end. Tho' I think I am an affable guy, I can't help wondering how I will behave when my dementia gets worse. And I wonder how much the memory problems are compounded by the natural aging process. I'll soon be eighty-three. I still have the curiosity of an old newsman.

13

I Forget More Names— but Not the People

Published April 11, 2015

You may remember in an earlier column I said that we intended to prepare our basement for a time when we might need live-in care. It now includes a renovated bedroom, a new, larger window, shelving, and a clothes closet. Outside the bedroom is a large room with a built-in desk, a counter to accommodate a kettle and toaster, and a short hallway to a full bathroom near remodelled stairs to the kitchen. A washer, dryer, and fridge will be shared.

Dorothea was lucky to find Doug and his crew, who were skilled and pleasant to have around. She worked closely with them because she knew exactly what she wanted. Considering the age of the house, it all worked out quite well.

In the meanwhile, of course, the space will be wonderful for visitors.

In January, I wrote about the arrangements Dorothea and I made with the bank to limit my access to funds. Now we learn from a news story about two wives of men with dementia who took issue with the actions of financial institutions that provided their husbands with what were called "irrational financial transactions." One was more severe than the other. In one case, the husband cashed in his life insurance for less than $2,000. On his death, it would pay $140,000. The other man bought a new car he didn't need, without consulting family. The wives of the men had the decisions of the institutions changed after some considerable, troubling efforts.

Neither man consulted his wife and, in one case, had not given his wife power of attorney.

I am not sure that on my own I would have thought of limits to my access so soon after my diagnosis, while I was still mentally active. We made our arrangements with the bank and the lawyer when I was able to participate fully. Fortunately, I still can.

The day we were given the news, we agreed that I should stop driving. That's a bit of a nuisance with only one driver in the family. But it made sense, and it seems to work all right.

As they say where I come from, I'm still hanging in there—reading newspapers and books, watching documentaries and other programs on television, and spending time with wonderful friends. However, I do have more memory loss. To deal with it, I keep a notebook near my den chair and by my computer. I jot down reminders. I have some difficulty with complicated instructions, but I may have an excuse. My dear mother, long gone, used to describe me as a "flockaholic omadhaun" when I was young. (See the *Dictionary of Newfoundland English* by George Story. The words mean about the same—I seldom took things seriously.)

Perhaps my difficulty with instructions is because I don't read them carefully. I now read my outgoing emails a few times before I hit the send button. And on more occasions, I forget names. However, forgetting someone's name does not mean forgetting who the person is. I don't feel embarrassed by that. It seems I have already let the cat out of the bag about my dementia.

Although my dementia has caused problems within the family, we've been fortunate. The mother of a close friend of ours was diagnosed with dementia when she was in her fifties, younger than my friend is now. I can't compare our situation with that of my friend's. This explains, I guess, why there'll be no *de profundis clamavi* from me. I seem to think I am becoming more needy. I'm sure I will be apprised if and when it surfaces.

A few years ago, on the suggestion of family, I wrote the story of my life. I wrote it in bits and pieces over several years while I was still working. My son, Peter, had hardcover copies printed for family, grandchildren, and some friends. I always regretted I knew so little about my grandparents' past, even though my father's parents lived next door or with us for some years. When I was my grandchildren's age, and long after, I never wondered and I never asked. I hope our grandchildren will get curious enough sometime to read their granddad's story.

After all, it includes their Nana Dorothea's story as well. We started dating when she was seventeen and I was twenty-three. I'm now closing in on eighty-three. The last page captures my diagnosis.

I had quite an interesting working life with wonderful jobs that I never thought I'd have, most of them in radio and television with CBC. I worked in four provinces and, for some months, with the UN in New York. I travelled to twenty countries. I once had lunch with Prime Minister John Diefenbaker, just the two of us, and I had a chance to chat with Jimmy Carter in Peru, of all places.

I ended my working career when I was seventy-five, as Nova Scotia's first freedom of information review officer. All on a grade 12 education. Not bad for a flockahoolic omadhaun!

I don't know how long I will be able to continue writing about my dementia. I think I'll know, or my family will. I don't want the editor of [the *Chronicle Herald*] left with the unpleasant job of telling me I'm past my due date. I think I'm still doing OK.

14

Life Goes on in Familiar Ways

Published September 15, 2015

"Our compassion recedes as their dementia advances. Memory, we believe, gives life its structure." These words were written by a *Globe and Mail* columnist in June. He was caring for his stepfather who, among other things, was demanding the car keys, even after he was found driving the wrong way on the highway to get his daughter at the airport. His daughter was not arriving.

For the writer, he admits it was easier to view his stepfather as a "lost cause." John Allemang said that he changed his mind after reading *The Theft of Memory* by Jonathan Kozol. A noted Boston neurologist whose father had dementia, Kozol wrote: "I loved my father. He was one of the most interesting people I have ever known, and I wanted to know him as well as I could, right to the end." I've read there are more than 740,000 Canadians living with some form of dementia, and that number will double by 2031. A book called *The Brain's Way of Healing* has been a bestseller for weeks. The author, Dr. Norman Doidge, admits that neurology was once considered a depressing discipline, with patients often displaying fascinating but essentially untreatable symptoms. Now, after thirty years of research, Doidge challenges that view using vivid portraits of patients and their physicians. A reviewer describes the book as "a treasure trove of the author's own deep insights and a clear bright light of optimism shines through every page." That "clear bright light of optimism" can be found in the eyes of Steve Patterson and Suzanne Daniels and their technician, Ron, at the IWK Health Centre in Halifax. I have now ended my tests at their neuroimaging research centre for which I was asked to volunteer—three two-hour sessions over thirty days. It ended with a fifteen-minute MRI.

During the sessions, I was "locked" into a huge fridge-like box with myriad wires attached to me and some sort of helmet over my head. It felt like I was in a tomb! Not really, though. I could hear and speak to those outside. A screen was pulled forward for me to watch images, and triggers were put in my hands. I was shown pictures and asked to identify them as living things or objects—one trigger for objects and the other for living things.

Steve and I fell out over one of my responses. He maintained that a strawberry was a living thing. I argued that because it was already picked, it was no longer living because it was removed from its source of life, the bush. It was dead, but edible, I maintained. Neither of us conceded but we enjoyed the argument. That was the tone set at these tests. In fact, I really enjoyed the entire exercise.

The curiosity of an old journalist, I suppose.

The tests ended with a chat with Suzanne, who asked some personal questions. My wife, Dorothea, joined us and kept me on track. I also had some questions for Suzanne, of course. No surprise there. I guess no marks were afforded for the tests...or I failed.

Some time later, local television did a story on dementia studies at the IWK. The reporter asked Suzanne if a "patient" would agree to an interview. She turned me in and I was happy to oblige.

Steve and Suzanne now need to find financing for further study. Of all the many worthy things people, through their governments, should finance, these studies should be near the top of the list.

Meanwhile, as I sat relaxed on a plane heading off to visit long-time friends in Toronto, I picked up the *Chronicle Herald* to learn that the biggest problem for the government that day was people like me who have the bad grace to live too long. I was one day shy of my eighty-third birthday. I felt everyone on the plane was staring at me. If the bad news is people living too long, what does it say about an old man with dementia? Perish the thought.

The government functionary giving us the bad news spoke in terms of available beds. More recently, my own CBC, where I spent forty years or more, allowed as how we old ones are really creating unprecedented problems for society. That being said, I have been paying taxes for more than sixty years and still do. And I'll hang on to my bed.

In Toronto, we went to the famous downtown market and got tangled up in a busload of older people. When the tour guides began to shepherd the elders back on the bus, Dorothea and I ducked to safety.

In an earlier column, I talked about our decision to put a hundred-dollar limit on my bank card lest I lose it or it's stolen. As luck should have it, I went into a Toronto bank at Dorothea's request to take out a few hundred dollars. When I inserted the card, the screen told me, rudely, that there was a hundred-dollar limit on it. Of course, I forgot that, and so did Dorothea when she sent me off.

A bank employee noticed my frustration and asked if she could help. I explained the problem and told her I had never had that problem before. She took me to the counter and instructed the teller to provide me with the few hundred dollars and off I went. Neither of us can understand how I got the money we wanted on my "flagged" card. I guess I beat the system.

(It has occurred to me that some readers may find all of this irrelevant, and I suppose it is. I guess I'm just trying to demonstrate that, after a diagnosis like mine, life can be pretty normal and very interesting and even provide lots of laughs.) So how am I doing? More names are escaping me. Recently, we drove to Wileville, near Bridgewater, NS, to visit friends who run a large market. When we got home, I forgot the name of the community but not the names of our friends. As it happens, one of them has the last name Wile.

However, I am still engaged in what we call current events and will certainly be making an informed choice in the next election. I'm still irreverent and somewhat brash and still reading two newspapers a day, several magazines a week, with a book by my chair. But I'm more likely to reread my emails before clicking on the send button.

There are days, of course, when I wonder how long I will be able to write about my dementia, or when life will no longer be "pretty normal." But there's still lots of humour in our house. The other day I spotted a book I wasn't sure I had read. So I picked it up and started reading. Halfway through, some of it looks familiar but some of it doesn't.

Dorothea joked that I could get by with two books from now on. Read two, forget the first one, and start that book again when I've finished the second one. By that time, the second book will have been forgotten.

I have agreed to volunteer for everything I have been asked to. Recently, I lent my name to a Dementia Friends program in Ottawa that is working closely with the Alzheimer Society of Canada. The developers of the program are planning to produce a video providing a quick snapshot of what it means to have dementia. As it happens, the woman who approached me is the granddaughter of a guy I knew who worked with the CBC years ago. I also agreed to be interviewed for television to speak on the work being done at the IWK. And I'll participate later this year in a Halifax panel on Alzheimer's and aging.

We stopped at the market in Masstown, NS, recently for lunch. Across from me was an elderly gentleman wearing a dress suit, stiff shirt, and tie with a fancy clasp. As Dorothea and I were leaving, I approached him with a smile, to suggest he was overdressed. He and his wife laughed, and she told me he always wears a suit when he goes out and has been doing so since he returned from the Second World War. He is ninety-three.

He complained to me that his wife filled bags with some eighty of his suits because, for decades, he has never been able to get rid of them. He told me some terrifying war stories before we left. I've learned you meet some wonderful and interesting people if you have the temerity to approach them. His wife told me he is also experiencing dementia and she thanked me for approaching him. Too many of us find it awkward to approach such "elders." His wife was grateful that I stopped to chat with him, though I had never seen him before that day.

I'm pleased that my dementia story has attracted the attention of people here in Nova Scotia, across the country, and even beyond.

This has encouraged me to continue writing about my experience for as long as I can.

15

A Trip Home Inspires Pleasant Memories

Published October 31, 2015

I am now adorned with a fancy engraved silver bracelet, the Medic Alert kind.

On it is engraved "Darce, Alzheimer's" and numbers to call. I have to confess; it is sobering to think that this bracelet will be on me from now on.

On a recent visit "home" to St. John's, I had even more sobering moments visiting my sister, Margaret, who has advanced dementia aggravated by a stroke. She has been in a care home in St. John's for several years. She is eighty-nine, the oldest of six children. I was the second-youngest. We are the only two left. One of my three brothers died with advanced Alzheimer's. The two other brothers died well before my age. My younger sister had Down syndrome and died in her forties. And there we are, two remaining, and both with dementia.

At the home where my sister is, Dorothea and I would walk past dozens of dementia patients, most of them in wheelchairs, to chat with Margaret. She usually recognized us, but not on every visit. It's no surprise that Dorothea, a good friend of my sister, is wonderful in situations like this, but I must confess it was somewhat daunting for me, as one might expect. Some patients would talk to us. Others were silent, and some were occasionally calling out, perhaps to no one.

Some days were better than others when we visited. At times, I would try to remind my sister of our days growing up at 50 Mullock

Street. To get her reaction, we brought a beautiful sweater she knit for me years ago. She felt it and said, "I did a good job." She had grasped a memory.

On one of our visits, a patient wheeled his chair over to ask if I knew "the Fardys from Flower Hill." I did know the Fardys from Flower Hill, first cousins. Another gentleman asked if he could come with us as we left.

Margaret has a wonderful friend, Sadie, a retired nurse, who visits her regularly. Margaret has no family in St. John's. Sadie is a godsend, as are the nurses and other caregivers at the home.

We still enjoy ourselves, and we live our lives to the full. And there's humour, lots of it.

We had taken the ferry to Argentia for the two-week visit to Newfoundland. While walking in North Sydney as we waited for the ferry, a woman we didn't know approached us to say how smart we looked for an older couple. I offered her a hug and she agreed with alacrity. Another woman was walking by, so I asked her if she wanted a hug and, of course, she did.

I'm wandering off topic. I usually do. In St. John's, I took many "memory walks" past the two houses my parents, grandparents, three brothers, and two sisters lived in when we were young. I remembered a lot about the neighbourhood. I also walked through the cavernous basilica, remembering my years as an altar boy and an attendant to the archbishop.

For some reason, I find walking alone and thinking to be almost curative.

Sometimes, to exercise my downgraded mind, I try a bit of math. An ad in the paper announced I could have a new car for so much down and so much a week for two or three years. I sharpened my pencil, so to speak, and had a shot at how much it would cost. I struggled a while and then mused, "To hell with it—we'll keep the trusty not rusty car we have." I surrendered, but I was always weak in math.

The federal election, of course, grabbed my full attention and held it. I watched until it was declared, and the next morning waited for the newspapers to read the election-night story. On politics, I'm a junkie. In my early days as a reporter with the CBC, I covered several elections in Newfoundland.

I discovered I no longer listen well to instructions. It seems I have abdicated. I've concluded that if Dorothea understands the instructions we are given, I don't need to. Perhaps I just have a lazy mind, but maybe there's more to it than that. I've pledged to listen to instructions more carefully.

We drove about 2,200 kilometres on our trip. Dorothea had to do all the driving. I provided comic relief. We both wonder if that was our final driving vacation back home.

I have a story to share involving grandson Seamus MacInnes, who told me recently that the photograph being used with my columns did not reflect reality. "Most pictures," he wrote, "make you look very serious and grumpy and without emotion, which is far from the case."

He said I looked in despair, staring vacantly, when in fact I'm still engaged and funny. The next day, the *Chronicle Herald* called to ask if they could come and take new photographs. The paper and Seamus probably reached that conclusion at the same time.

Seamus, who is seventeen, recently wrote in a grade 12 assignment about his granddad's approach to dementia: "Instead of letting it define him, he tries to define dementia." Can't beat a tribute like that! I am proud that Dorothea and I decided to make the grandchildren aware of what's going on.

So how am I doing? Besides opting out of listening to instructions, I have been repeating questions, sometimes within half an hour after I uttered the first one. Most of the time I realize what I've done. My attention wanders, I guess.

Recently, someone mentioned Mumford Road; I couldn't remember where it was. In fact, we drive Mumford Road several times a week for shopping and the drugstore.

Just as I'm sorting out the new realities, our Mayor Mike decides it's time to reorganize curbside collection and make substantial changes. All of my neighbours appeared confused and huddled together to ask questions. Most of them seem to have a handle on it now. Me? Not so much.

I usually put the garbage out with my fingers crossed that no bags will be refused. I'm still struggling. And to think that as an altar boy I could recite the entire mass in Latin. Now I can't even put my mind to the garbage instructions. *Mea culpa!*

Back to reality. Dorothea and I have volunteered for other Alzheimer's tests, this time with True North Clinical Research, which offers free testing. Another opportunity to help the cause of research into dementia.

I've been thinking recently of the stress families are under when one member is no longer able to live at home. In my next column, I hope to address that. I want to leave some guidance to my family, in their favour and mine.

2016

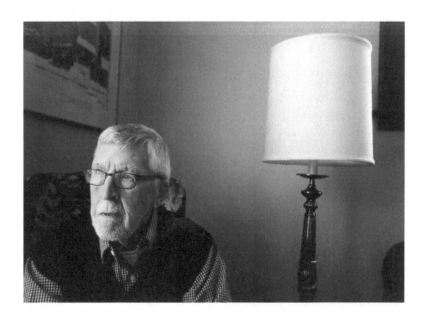

16

Moderate Memory Lapses and a Focus on Current Events

Published January 2, 2016

Dementia creeps, and the search continues to find a way to reverse the creep.

This Christmas was the third since I was diagnosed and hopefully someday scientists and researchers will get a handle on it. And that explains my willingness to participate in Alzheimer's research whenever I can.

My experience shows it's a slow creep. Later, I suppose, it could become a jog.

Dorothea and I have volunteered to take part in a four-year study of dementia. The testing, at True North Clinical Research in Halifax, includes direct memory questions from one of the professionals at the clinic. As an example, Dana, a memory therapist at the clinic, would ask me to listen to eight words and to repeat them in order. He used common, unrelated words: "board," "shepherd," "carrot," "suitcase," "desk," "tree," "bulb," "table." I didn't get many right.

Questions became more complex throughout that session. The responses need to be analyzed by an expert, not by me, so I won't try. But I did score myself very low on some. Dana remained strenuously non-judgmental when I asked how I performed. He learned quickly I was a curious guy. I probably put as many questions to him as he did to me. And he obliged.

I was curious to see images of brains with and without dementia.

He left the room and found one. I concluded that the brain showing the most "matter" was the brain without dementia. I was wrong, and when he explained, it made sense.

After the questionnaire, I was given a physical exam by Rikki and then by Dr. Mark. Both were professional, with a good sense of humour. That's a must for me.

During all this, Dorothea was in an adjoining room answering questions, presumably about my behaviour at home. A sneaky manoeuvre, perhaps. She told me later she heard a lot of chatter from me next door.

So far, so pretty good.

I am encouraged by emails, cards, and comments, often from people I don't know, to continue writing about my experience for as long as I can, as long as the *Chronicle Herald* has room for it.

Recently, I was looking through bookshelves in a store when a woman approached to ask if I were the man who was writing the columns in the newspaper. Another woman approached me at the farmers' market. And a supermarket employee approached Dorothea and asked if the man with her was the guy who wrote the articles.

I also received a wonderful card expressing appreciation for my decision to go public. I know that some people are loath to approach me, and I urge them not to hesitate. Most have family dementia issues of their own. I was told by one woman, now a friend, that her father was at a point where he couldn't remember the name of one of his children. I'm told by friends who visit that I show no signs of dementia. But there are signs, and in my house, we are well aware of them.

But my problems are moderate so far. Names elude me more but sometimes for only a few minutes. Recent memory lapses include not remembering a decision we made on what to give one of our daughters for Christmas (that concerned me) and forgetting the names of people only hours after I spent the afternoon with them. I know, of course, who they were, though I hadn't seen them in about forty years. The names always return, perhaps moments later. I fear that later I will be losing names even of people close to me. I don't want to think about that.

Minor lapses are fairly easy to hide. Recently, I went shopping with Dorothea and daughter Donna to buy some family Christmas gifts. I quickly realized I was in a ladies' shoe store, and that this purchase could take longer than any man would expect. So I wandered off to see if any other store would capture my interest. None did, so I returned to the shoe store, and I wandered past it. I made it back before a search began.

When I tell stories like that about myself, I will often get the reply, "That happens to me many times." And perhaps it does. And perhaps passing this store was like that...or not.

All of this, you will agree, is minor, except if you have dementia. That said, during the recent federal election campaign, I captured it all. I'm a political junkie and have been since the days of Louis St. Laurent, John Diefenbaker, Joey Smallwood, and Tommy Douglas. And the December attack on Paris dominated my interest for days, as does the Syrian refugee issue.

Dorothea and I read two newspapers a day and pick up the freebies when passing the sidewalk boxes, and we talk about what we read.

I remain concerned that my condition, as it advances, will preoccupy my family when/if I move out of my home and into care. I want my daughters and son and my daughter-in-law, Carol, to be preoccupied with their own families.

I have a bit of an advantage in Carol. She's a nurse, and good nurses like Carol can be professional and practical as well as compassionate. She will be a good connection between the family and nurses and aides. And we love her.

I am not being noble when I say I worry more about how this affects my family than I do about myself. I'll be eighty-four in May, which, perversely, is kind of good news. It's a morbid thought, but I could die from other causes before I slip gently into the fog of dementia. I have done more than I ever hoped to in my life and had more satisfying jobs than I ever expected or planned for. That said, while I'd like to go before my dementia sets in, I'm not ready yet, because I still enjoy life.

I continue to test myself. I recently read Lawrence Hill's *The Illegal*. I'd put it down for a day or so in a deliberate attempt to determine if I could remember what I'd read when I picked it up again. In it, Hill writes about what he terms "living without dignity or autonomy." He wasn't writing about Alzheimer's, but it fits.

Meanwhile, *Zoomer*, a magazine for us oldies, muses that there may soon be a time when cancer and Alzheimer's are just a nuisance. Not in my time, but let the research continue and let our governments support it.

A prominent man who died recently, former British Columbia premier Bill Bennett, was described as having struggled "with" Alzheimer's. He may have died "with" dementia/Alzheimer's, but did he die "from" it? That's a question I'd like answered.

As an aside, I am also seized with finding some indication that the prescribed pills I take are helping. I find they can sometimes be quite unfriendly. True North's Dana should prepare for more questions when next we meet.

Finally, daughter Donna sent me a story containing the results of a study done by the American Society's *Journal of Agriculture and Food Chemistry* proclaiming that beer can be helpful for those with dementia. I also hear red wine may be beneficial.

Now if I could persuade them to have a look at Manhattans and get the same result, then we're talking.

17

A Humbling Christmas Face Plant

Published January 30, 2016

There are now an estimated 17,000 of us in Nova Scotia, according to the reckoning of the Alzheimer Society of Nova Scotia. And I expect we are all different, in our own ways. And what's my way? How is my mind functioning? I spend a lot of time trying to examine my own mind. A fool's errand perhaps.

I think I'm more and more frustrated by my inability to do things I had always done with ease: recording television programs, playing discs and the like. Or perhaps my mind is getting lazy because I don't insist on doing all that. I'm on Facebook, but I've never used it and I don't intend to. Recently, the family set up Netflix and Apple TV for us. I watched from the sideline. I have to get a handle on all that stuff quickly.

When you offer to go public with your dementia, you are obliged, of course, to be truthful and open and as complete as possible.

A week before Christmas, I took a tumble on a hard sidewalk. I guess you'd call it a face plant. It left me scarred and humbled. For the first time in eighty-three years, I felt fragile. I suppose it was related to my dementia one way or another, but we don't know. What I do know is that I didn't slip on ice.

I fell while walking to daughter Donna's home. I was a few houses away when I suddenly fell face-first to the sidewalk. I was unhurt but unable to get up without help. Fortunately, two women came along to try to help. I couldn't see them as they struggled to get me up. I heard one of them say she would fetch her husband. He managed to get me up and walked me to my daughter's house. I didn't know the damage until I saw Donna's reaction when she opened the door—my face was pretty banged up.

Later, like a good neighbour would, the Good Samaritan returned to Donna's house to see how I was. He applied a few physical tests, prompting Donna to ask if he were a doctor. He is an accountant, but as luck should have it he is also an emergency ski slope guy. He has probably handled some great tumbles. To continue a tale even Ripley couldn't embrace, his wife is an emergency room nurse. Fortunately, I didn't need his wife's skills, but it was a good spot to drop.

At a walk-in clinic, the doctor checked me out and I went home with the hope the scars would be gone before our Christmas party.

It was, I guess, the most embarrassing moment of my long life. I've done a lot of dumb stuff in my years, but that one takes the cake. From the time I was diagnosed with dementia, I was advised to use a cane because there could be some moments of instability. And I do; I had it in hand when I fell. In this case, it happened so suddenly and unexpectedly the cane was no help.

So I'm out of the Christmas photos and will be under more family scrutiny, at least for the remainder of the winter. I'll sulk about it, for sure.

On a more positive note, I received a wonderful email recently:

> I have been reading your articles in the *Chronicle Herald* and must say I admire your ability to captain your own journey. My father was diagnosed about five years ago with vascular dementia and then Lewy body dementia, but the name doesn't really matter, I quickly realized. My dad, like you, is much more than that.
>
> His journey takes its own path, and each turn has been difficult, but he is always so graceful. A source of strength really for the rest of us! As strange as it sounds

as change comes, my dad is still the same. You are so right about having a nurse in the family! My mom has been invaluable to not only my dad but to the rest of us.

The phrase "captain your own journey" struck a note with me. I guess that's what I'm doing, with Dorothea as first officer and my family as the crew. This ship would sink without them.

I am still being stopped in stores by people telling me my columns have helped them understand what's happening in their families. Often the concern is that the member of their family with dementia is still driving. That issue arose when I was diagnosed. I quit immediately, but I have a driver's licence and will drive in an emergency. As it happened, before there was any sign of dementia, Dorothea and I decided to take driver's tests just to ensure we were still up to scratch. One of us scored higher than the other, but I won't boast about that.

Quitting cold turkey, as I did, is not easy. It's very difficult because you feel grounded and dependent, even if there is another driver in the family. But I am convinced it is the thing to do for everyone's safety.

18

The Movie about a Nursing Home Was Hard to Watch

Published February 20, 2016

When you're living with someone with dementia there is always concern that kitchen stoves may be left on, empty kettles plugged in, and the like.

We had a visit since my last column from a man who is searching for ways to keep those with dementia living safely in their own homes. He told us he was inspired to do this by his mother's actions in her home when she lived alone. On two occasions ambulances arrived at her house because of a misdirected telephone call.

Beyond doctoring the telephone, improvements could include some changes to the buttons on stoves, microwaves, and thermostats. Changes could be made to allow access only to radio and television programs that the person with dementia enjoys. This gentleman has an urge to work on such changes and came to ask Dorothea and me for any comments. We wish him well.

Although there is no cure for dementia yet, researchers are, thankfully, continuing to test the effectiveness of drugs in slowing down the advance of the disease or—who knows?—curing it. It encourages me to continue making myself available to be poked and prodded by researchers.

I volunteered for a PET scan recently and the researcher who organized it reported back that my dementia is confirmed in the scan. (I'm hoping I can see the scan and compare it with a scan of a person without dementia.) Researchers hope tests like mine may help them find a cure someday. Not in my time, of course, but there is always hope. I have two more sessions coming up: one with a dermatologist, and another, a three-hour session at True North Clinical Research.

I had never heard of the movie *Wrinkles* when I was invited to join a panel to view the movie with an audience. *Wrinkles* is an animated film based on a comic of the same name. It is centred in a home for the aging and begins with a son losing patience with his absent-minded father and deciding he should be in care. The film features men and women and their activities and behaviour at the home.

Wrinkles and another film which ran in theatres called *Still Alice* were shown to the public as part of Alzheimer's month. Many people are familiar with *Still Alice*.

Joining me on the panel to discuss *Wrinkles* were a geriatrician, a psychiatrist, and an epidemiologist. I was described as a "journalist and patient advocate"...three learned panel members out of four ain't bad. It was moderated by Tim Krahn, a research associate at Dalhousie Medical School. The audience asked questions after the screening. As someone with dementia, I expected to be asked what my conclusions were after watching the movie.

Dorothea and daughter Donna were there for the event. Parts of the movie can be difficult for families with dementia in their midst. I viewed the film at home three times with Dorothea before the public screening. I wanted to find out how we both would react. My reaction was emotional, hers was analytical. I was glad our views were different. She saw value in the movie, and I saw little even after a third viewing. But I hung in.

There are parts that provoked laughter among those attending the screening. But the laughter was muted and didn't last long. I suppose those laughing suddenly felt guilty.

I think the session was helpful, well arranged, and worthwhile. The people attending were anxious to find out what the panel members had to offer, and it was a lot. I think having a panel member with dementia offered the audience a unique opportunity to pose some questions to me.

Viewing the movie for the fourth time didn't change my original reaction. I found it difficult to watch and disturbing, with little value. But that may have been my reaction alone. And there are funny moments.

I'd like to tell you about the afternoon Dorothea and I spent with the young woman whose email to me I quoted from in my last column. I searched her out through her email address to have a chat. I discovered she lived nearby. We suggested she drop by for a cup of tea. Meeting in a crowded café didn't seem to be the place to chat. She agreed, of course, and we met on a Sunday afternoon, comfy in our living room with the fireplace on. It was a wonderful experience for the three of us.

Julia is a young teacher in Halifax. Her father, mother, and other siblings live in Saint John, NB, and she visits regularly. During her visit there was lots of laughter and a tear from time to time when she spoke of her dad, who has a more difficult dementia than I do. The three of us enjoyed the session and will certainly stay in touch and remain friends.

We got a lot of feedback from my last column, all of them encouraging me to keep writing my columns and I will, given the "creek don't rise" and [the *Chronicle Herald*] continues to publish them.

Meanwhile, we all know that aging brings a bundle of new problems. Dementia brings even more problems. I'm amazed we manage so well. Recently, I met up with Tim, an old colleague at the CBC years and years ago. Although he is four or five years older than I am and tells me he also has dementia, he recognized me. But I couldn't capture his name. Dorothea came by and recognized him immediately. Tim had an advantage, of course, because he read my columns.

At the supermarket lineup recently the man ahead of me came back after checking out to ask if I were Darce Fardy. He suspected I couldn't remember his name and he offered it. I did remember him as a CBC broadcaster a long, long time ago.

Okay, so how am I doing otherwise? I'm forgetting more, though only for a moment or two. When the former broadcaster asked me where I lived, I replied, "The Danforth." That avenue, of course, is in Toronto, where I lived for several years. I have no idea what brain cell provided that answer. I quickly amended it and he didn't comment. I guess he reads my columns.

To leave you on a lighter tone, one of Justin Trudeau's promises during last year's campaign was to amend the Elections Act. I understand the present system but am wrestling with the proposed one. All of this despite the fact I covered politics and elections for a number of years. I guess I'll have to invite Dan Leger, a first-class political observer, out for a bowl of soup and ask him to explain it slowly.

19
Parliament Should Consult Canadians on End of Life

Published March 12, 2016

hen preparing this column, I intended to go where angels fear to tread to the issue of assisted living/dying. But Parliament beat me to it. Suddenly the gates opened when we learned that a special Parliamentary committee will propose that Parliament debate a new physician-assisted dying law that includes advance consent from people in early stages of dementia.

There's been a motherlode of media attention given to dementia/ Alzheimer's recently, even before the announcement of the parliamentary committee.

Assisted living/assisted dying is the crux of a recent public discussion. A columnist in the *Globe and Mail*, Andre Picard, wrote a column headed, "A Dignified Death for Dementia Patients: Who Makes the Call?" It was Picard's column that encouraged me to consider the options. It is, of course, a controversial moral and legal issue and I have been giving it some thought. I want to make the decision with my family. They will know explicitly what I want when I am no longer able to contribute to the discussions. Then I want my family to make the decision when I should be left to die or assisted to die. It's a burden on them for sure, but at least they will know what I want. If I have already "faded to black," as we used to say in television, but still alive, they will be able to let me go. I expect my family doctor will help the family understand the process.

Picard's column inspired a number of letters to the editor. In one of them a writer said his father had requested "as quick an end as possible" if he were no longer "capable of rational existence." Another writer believes "the right to vote one's own conscience on a matter of such fundamental importance lies at the very heart of liberal democracy."

I thought about all of this a while ago when Dorothea and I visited my ninety-year-old sister in a long-term care home in St. John's. She has been there ten years with no hope of a cure. She appears to be in constant torment. So is it appropriate to give her medication, for example, for high blood pressure to prolong her life?

I am learned in neither the law nor theology so I'm in a place now where angels fear to tread. But I'm no angel and my knowledge of the law compares with my knowledge of the solar system.

A close friend and law professor is helping me navigate the intricacies of the law and lead[ing] me safely through the jungle of my thoughts on the issues raised in the media. Wayne MacKay pointed out there is an important distinction between asking that doctors refrain from doing things (no revival by heroic means or prolonging a life) and asking doctors to actively assist in dying by administering medications (assisted death).

Clarity is needed on what is wanted—active or passive intervention. It's a complex family issue but, given my age and the futility of expecting a cure in my time, I favour active. I pray that with all of the hard work being done by researchers around the world that my family, including my grandchildren and theirs, will not have to deal with dementia.

I will be eighty-four in a few weeks and I'm still enjoying myself and not imposing too much of a burden on Dorothea or the rest of my family. But a decline is inevitable. We will have a family chat as we try to address this problem and take advantage of new thinking.

Increasingly, the Supreme Court is seen as Canada's main policy-maker, but it's now down to the politicians to pass the laws.

We are told parliamentarians have discussed the issue. There are likely hundreds of people who have been diagnosed and are where I am today. I hope members of the Commons will consult with all Canadians, particularly with those who have been diagnosed but can still contribute. I am one of those. This is all such a personal family issue that having legislators discussing it among themselves would not be enough. I hope those who want to have input in the discussion will contact their member of Parliament.

Chantal Hébert, one of my favourite newspaper columnists, said in [the *Chronicle Herald*] that there's evidence the members of the House of Commons may put divisive debating aside and support [medical assistance in dying]. Having watched Parliament in action I can't help but be concerned.

The report also calls on the federal government to work with the provinces and territories to make medically assisted dying available. Let's hope that will happen.

20

I'm Starting to Forget a Few Things Now

Published April 23, 2016

Hope blooms. More promising news on Alzheimer's. As reported in [the *Chronicle Herald*], after twenty years of studies, a group of researchers in Halifax have made a world-leading breakthrough in early Alzheimer's detection.

To help in any small way, Dorothea and I continue our volunteer work at a clinic engaged in trying to find a cure for the disease. We are signed up for a four-year study. On our latest visit we were both interviewed separately by the staff of True North. I learned later that Dorothea, in her own session, was asked about our recent activities in and outside the house. Some of that information was used in a subsequent interview with me to determine if I could remember and comment. For example, they were told by Dorothea about a movie we saw recently and how much we both enjoyed it. When they asked me about it later, I remembered seeing the movie but not the name of the movie or the name of the famous English star or even the name of the theatre. But I did remember the movie. So I guess I didn't strike out. On our way home from the clinic I remembered the answer to all three questions and was tempted to rush back to the clinic to announce: "I got it."

Usually, from time to time, I like to share how I'm doing. I am certainly forgetting more. I may be asking Dorothea the same question a few times and forgetting the answer in the end. Recently, we went with friends to Peggys Cove, where there are cottages and a wonderful restaurant. I had driven there myself before and now I couldn't remember the way. Later, we drove Dorothea's visiting brother, Doug, to the Chester/Lunenburg area to sightsee and have lunch. When we got back, I was asked by my daughter where we had gone and I couldn't grab the names of the towns we drove through.

I'm still doing okay writing my columns, but I can't type like I used to. I have been at a keyboard since I was a young journalist sixty years ago. Never a "touch typist," but close. Not anymore, though. Now I'm almost back to the "hunt and peck" way. I have to proofread the column again and again, as does Dorothea. I do remember the spelling of words even if I don't always strike the right keys.

I decided to recharge the batteries on my camera in advance of a crowded Easter dinner with the extended family. I have done it dozens of times. This time it was challenging. On the upside, I don't have to hide my memory problems. Most everyone knows, and my offences are venial. I also put the wrong kind of soap in the dishwasher and soap bubbles began escaping. All of this a few days before a large family Easter dinner. I wouldn't categorize this as a venial error!

Recently, we were invited to meet the organizers of Hospice Halifax, a first for Nova Scotia. Two large homes will be joined to prepare a place for patients to spend their final days. Briefly, a hospice provides a place to die in comfort and relative privacy, tended to by health professionals. I understand it will be only the second one in the Atlantic Provinces. Patients would have their own room where families could gather around in peace and quiet to say goodbye. Large windows would bring in the sun. I understand it will be one of only two such hospices in Atlantic Canada.

Pets are invited to come with their visiting family. I'm guessing the visiting pets don't include snakes or squirrels...and the dogs are expected to behave. Dorothea and I were invited to meet the wonderful group of volunteers in one of the two large houses that will form the hospice. And we were interviewed together for our reaction. We were impressed by the energy and passion of the volunteers and the plans they have. (Hospice Halifax has a website.)

As we were driving our grandson David, our youngest grandchild, home from school recently, he asked me what it was like to lose your memory. I'll try to work out some of the answers in my next column. I suspect frustration will be at the top of the list. It's a tough disease.

In other columns I spoke of my sister Margaret in a nursing home in St. John's for the past ten years. She died, mercifully, while I was writing this column. It was a few days before her ninetieth birthday. A gift and card were in the mail.

21

I Remember Dief the Chief, but Not the Local Eatery

Published May 14, 2016

What is it with memories, at least my memory?

I remember seeing Nikita Khrushchev banging his shoe on his desk at the United Nations General Assembly in 1960 in New York when I worked there. I remember watching Fidel Castro cruising through Manhattan standing in a Jeep; I remember trying to get an interview with Yuri Gagarin, the first man in space, when his flight (not his space flight) connected in Gander, NL.

I remember having dinner with John Diefenbaker in St. John's during an election campaign and chatting with Jimmy Carter in Lima, Peru, at a freedom of information conference. I remember the Queen's visit to St. John's, when the convertible she and the Prince were driving in broke down. He suggested buying British-made cars.

So how come I forget the name of a restaurant we favour?

I can still find my lapses amusing. Recently, I tried to contact Steve Murphy of CTV because we had shared an experience. As you would expect, I went to the CTV website to find his email address. I couldn't find it. I googled him without success.

So I found myself going to the Yellow Pages to find a telephone number for CTV. I found one, phoned the number, and connected with Steve. Then it struck my fancy: a journalist for forty years, I was left thumbing through the Yellow Pages to get to find Steve. I'm going to have to learn to tweet. I now try to rethink things I do automatically—did I close the fridge door, did I lock the front and back doors, did I turn off the lights? I approach the microwave with caution. Now, I suppose, I may be too careful, too hesitant.

When I don't get Bruce MacKinnon's scriptless political cartoons, then I'll know.

In my last column, I promised to address my grandson David's question: What's it like to lose your memory? The first word I come up with is "frustrating." Not "depressing," or "angry," or "in despair." I think you can conceal those thoughts. I don't think you can hide frustration. But for the most part I can hold the frustration at bay.

Dorothea and I continue our practice of watching British mysteries on television. I was always able to follow the plot, if not identify the culprit. Now I'm given to look to Dorothea for clarification, so we now record the shows and she can stop the program to explain what's happening.

Other noticeable lapses. I couldn't remember Tom Mulcair's name when television, radio, and newspapers were full of NDP leadership issues. Much more disturbing, of course, is if I don't remember the name of a grandchild. It happened recently for a few moments. It's awful.

On the brighter side, when I called my doctor's office to have Frank look at my sore foot, his wife, who was at the front desk, gave me a 3:00 P.M. appointment...and told me not to forget to bring my foot. That's the way I want it.

I have to say, I'm encouraged when people we don't know approach us. At the library recently, on three occasions, people came up to speak with us. I suspect they all have dementia in their families. Since my last column, Dorothea and I participated in a public forum on dementia put on by the Alzheimer Society of Nova Scotia. It was a wonderful event. Dozens of people chatted with us. I'll write about it in another column if the *Chronicle Herald* obliges.

Ten or more years ago, I began writing my story: from a patched-pants scruffian running around the unpaved Mullock Street in St. John's to a few years ago. Son, Peter, had hard-covered books produced with enough copies for all of my grandchildren. When I started *My Story*, it never occurred to me I'd be using it for research purposes for these columns. The final page reveals my diagnosis.

I got some encouragement listening to the *Sunday Morning* program on CBC Radio. They were talking about the doorway effect. Apparently, it is common for many to forget why they are at the door before entering a room. It concludes that's caused by a distraction, not by a memory lapse. I take comfort where I can.

22

Where Would We Be without Loved Ones?

Published June 17, 2016

True story. The phone rang the other day and daughter Donna, in a bit of a rush, asked me for my postal code number.

Immediately, I provided it. When I hung up, I asked myself, "How in heaven did I grasp that tiny little piece of memory?" I am amazed that somewhere in my crippled brain lay my postal code number, left unused in this day and age of emails (now becoming old-fashioned), texts, and tweets.

I told the story to great amusement. I'll have to ask my friends at the memory clinic, where I volunteer, to confirm that there is a part of the brain reserved to hold information not needed anymore...it just becomes more difficult to find.

Donna, by the way, assures me she wasn't testing me.

In a recent column, I promised to tell you about a wonderful forum organized by the local Alzheimer Society—Life Doesn't End When Dementia Begins. The forum was organized by Linda Bird, the Society's director of programs and services, and by other staff and many volunteers.

The meeting room appeared crowded, so I guess half of those attending had dementia and the other half are the wonderful people who "mind" them. The session started with Janet, the keynote speaker, telling us of her experience since she first noticed a change in Jack's behaviour and decided to check it out. An avid Rotarian, he had lost interest a few years back. His driving was erratic. Since the diagnosis was confirmed, they go for daily walks and go to the theatre in the afternoons. Janet prefers not to drive at night. Jack wears an ID bracelet.

It was Janet's advice that it might be helpful, when speaking to someone with dementia, to break a sentence in two parts. For example, you might ask that person to enter the living room and, once in, to then invite that person to sit down. Dorothea was the first to notice my lapses. Where would Jack and I and many others be without devoted partners or friends?

I was on a panel with Kara, Anne, and Tony. Kara is with the Society and helped organize the event. I suspect Kara was on the panel to make sure I gave others a chance to be heard. She had met me earlier over coffee. The panel was there to offer advice. We eschewed that in favour of telling our own stories.

Tony, I guess, has no spare time. He hikes tirelessly to keep body strong and spirits high. I was a little abashed by his regular exercises. I thought I heard him mention Everest, but I guess not.

Tony wears a tracking device when he's out on his own. I wear a Medic Alert bracelet carved with my name, my disease, Dorothea's cellphone number, and a hotline number. Anne lives alone. She has a close friend, on whom she depends, who accompanied her to the forum. Anne has calendars in different parts of the house and always carries a notebook with her. Her friend is never far away, I guess. I was so moved by Anne's remarks I couldn't resist giving her a hug.

One man attending the conference was in a later stage of dementia. He appeared agitated from time to time, standing up occasionally to look back, and at one time picking up his jacket. We learned he was looking for his son. When his son appeared, his agitation seemed to evaporate.

An occupational therapist spoke on brain changes, function, and tips for those who care for us. Carol Ann provided us with practical information, from memory strategies like marking important dates on a calendar, to placing keys in the same place, and decluttering cluttered spaces.

And Carol Ann suggests quiet times. That's the toughest suggestion for me to take. I wouldn't be good at "silent times."

As for my own trip down this road, I appear to be more tired in the morning than when I went to bed. I suspect there is a rogue pill among the many I take. My sleeps are restless. I must investigate. This means nagging the researcher at the clinic where Dorothea and I volunteer.

And now spring is here and we're planting tomatoes and sugar peas, hanging baskets, and reading our books on the deck. Our son, Peter, and daughter-in-law, Carol, have urged us to use their cottage in Northport and we try to get there whenever we can. It's a wonderful break after a cold (indoor) winter.

When Dorothea is asked how I'm doing, she says, "He's losing his memory, not his intellect."

23

Thank Goodness I Still Have a Sense of Humour

Published July 15, 2016

So, here's how it went down at our recent visit to the medical clinic where we help in its search for a cure for what I have. Dorothea was taken aside while I was shunted off to another area. She was asked a few questions:

Can your husband shop for, plan, and cook a meal? Her reply: Don't know!

Can he balance the budget? He's never had to.

Can he do the laundry? Same answer...Never has.

I usually clear up after meals and fill the dishwasher and empty it. Given the time I put in the wrong soap and started a mini-flood, I let my spouse start the dishwasher. She insists, in fact. I don't think I could have created a skit like that for a comedy show.

In my own admittedly weak defence, I need to explain that I travelled a lot during my years with the CBC and on two occasions I was away an entire year, with periodic visits home.

I spent a year with a few other civilians at the National Defence College in Kingston, ON, to better understand Canada's role in the world. [Select senior officers, senior public servants, and corporate executives spent a year travelling across Canada and to dozens of other countries to learn the history of geo-political and military issues between 1948 and 1994.–*Ed.*] With senior officers, we visited some of the countries we discussed. Although I was home occasionally, I thought better of involving myself, or even commenting on, prevalent procedures.

Later, as I was about to retire from the CBC, I was asked to stay for another twelve months. We had already sold our Toronto home, so I took an apartment and Dorothea came back to Halifax to house-hunt and move our furniture.

In all, we lived in two houses in St. John's, two in Halifax, and two in Toronto. We also spent a year in Edmonton, AB, but that didn't include buying a house.

She was kind enough, though, to send change-of-address notices. On at least one occasion, she finalized a house-buying while I was away. We have lived in five houses, in St. John's, Halifax, and Toronto. In Edmonton we made living arrangements.

Back to the clinic. The questions put to me tend to go on and on and on. Some of that is my fault because I can't resist asking my own questions. Whatever my answer to his question, the staffer says, "good" and goes on to the next questions. He's a cool guy and tries to ignore my own probing questions into what he's doing. I get a few more questions from other staff and get jabbed with the inevitable needle. I don't know why they do that, if not for the amusement of those who administer it.

All of this could take two hours. Dorothea suggests it could be shorter if I'd stop talking so much during the process.

Whatever, we are pleased to be involved.

We had a visitor recently, a close friend of Dorothea's. She and Sylvia talked about her son's wedding. I asked some questions and was told I [had been] there, what the weather was like, and so on, and so on, and so on. I don't remember the wedding, even after being told some of the specifics. I find I am forgetting "stuff" more and more.

We recently had two guests for dinner, one of them with a more advanced dementia than I have. I must confess it was awkward for me to talk to someone with issues I have yet to, but will, face.

But there is always humour. Dorothea was talking to a friend on the phone after that dinner and told her that our guest didn't even remember being in our home before. I broke up the conversation by shouting, "Neither do I." That provoked a healthy laughter and I hope we can have more and more of it.

But simpler and happier times always prevail. We watched a grandson and granddaughter graduate from high school at a wonderful ceremony. Then we all got together at Amber's house for a graduation party. Granddaughter Molly baked a cake and cookies for the event. I'm sure the cake and cookies made it to many Facebooks. Most of those attending were young women, all university students or graduates. Having contact with young, smart people is important to me and perhaps even important to them.

With Alzheimer's, you are not out of it until you are. But there remains a certainty. Sooner or later, I will not be here and if I am, I won't know I am.

There is a noticeable, slow decline and I will write about it in my next column if [the *Chronicle Herald*] obliges.

24

I Can't Remember My Address, but I Can Dance

Published August 5, 2016

I t happened, as I thought it would someday, but sooner than I'd hoped.

I took a cab recently to head home. As I opened the cab door, I couldn't remember my address. It was somewhere in a crevice of my damaged brain. So I took my time arranging my cane and then feigned having trouble with my seat belt. And then I grasped the address from that crevice and off we went.

Later, I wondered how the driver would have reacted if my search were unsuccessful. Of course, all that information was in my wallet, but it never occurred to me I would need it.

A few days later I took another cab, but this time I was ready. If I were walking home, I would not have had the problem. I know there will be more lapses as I navigate the unpredictable "mind" fields ahead. I have my moments, of course, but they are rare.

I'm inspired by my own family, Dorothea, Sheila, Donna, and Carol, who have all faced daunting experiences and have prevailed. I have many pleasant distractions with wonderful friends. And I'm eighty-four.

Before sending in this column, we spent a day with friends from Connecticut and an overnighter from two friends from Yellowknife. One of the distractions was a big party to celebrate Peter and

Carol's twenty-fifth wedding anniversary, held in the town hall in Northport, NS, where they have a cottage. Our entire family, grandchildren, and all, joined a crowd of friends who filled the hall.

As the oldest person there, I was probably the most active. I abandoned my cane and danced with any woman who would dance with me—daughters, grandchildren, and all. I even managed to coax my reluctant teenage granddaughter Molly to join me. Someone took a picture of us and I am convinced there was a smile. I also danced with six-foot granddaughter Gabrielle. I threatened she would be out of the will if she picked me up.

Dorothea sat bemused while I was showing off, but someone whispered the news to band leader Dale that it was our fifty-eighth wedding anniversary. So, Dale, out of due respect, slowed the beat down a bit and I took in my arms the girl I first dated when she was seventeen and danced a slow one, to the bemusement of the grandkids. Then Peter intercepted to take his mother and I hugged and danced with Carol. Band leader Dale is from Northport, and we encouraged his parents to come to the party. They did, and I danced with his mother. Linda and Owen are wonderful friends.

A reader may wonder what all this has to do with my struggle with my dementia.

The answer is it has everything to do with it! Life goes on and, with the help of family and many friends, we will prevail.

I still enjoy reading and just finished an autobiography of a former federal cabinet minister. And I still read my newspapers.

When Someone You Know Has Dementia is a new book Dorothea is reading. Heavy reading, I'm sure. Given my age, it is likely I will be gone before I reach the most difficult possibilities. Dorothea did not recommend I read it. It's meant for those who live with the person who has dementia, not, in her view, someone who has it.

Some time ago I reported in a speech to the Alzheimer Society that I had been banned from the marital bed. Some rogue pill was being unfriendly, and I tossed and turned a lot, so I am out in the other room. On a few mornings recently I turned in the bed and noticed Dorothea wasn't next to me. I was surprised she got up without waking me. She wasn't sleeping there, of course, and has never slept in the bed I inherited.

So, my practice remains to keep looking back. Looking forward is too predictable.

25

My Memory Is Fading More Quickly than I'd Hoped

Published September 2, 2016

Who would have thought that a birthday party would bring a significant challenge to my memory—the most significant challenge since I was diagnosed four years ago?

We were in Toronto to celebrate Christine's birthday. She and her husband, Bob, have been wonderful friends for years. And so has their extended family. Bob and I were together at the CBC for many years.

More than a few retired "CBC-ers" were at the party. And there the memory was challenged. I sometimes remembered the jobs these people had but not their names. I eventually chatted with all of them but at times forgot their names shortly after remembering them or even while I was talking to them. Most or all of the former CBC-ers were aware of my condition, so that made it easier. Of course, I would have told them anyway. I hadn't seen some of these people since I retired from the CBC twenty-five years ago.

Back home I was sent out to the corner store recently for milk and one of their delicious sandwiches which we often have. I got the milk, picked up a candy bar, and forgot the sandwich. After I paid and was about to leave, I remembered the sandwich. The owner knows about my memory loss and figured I forgot the sandwich but didn't want to remind me in case I didn't want one.

We laughed, but other customers must have wondered. One reason, I guess, for forgetting the sandwich is that I bought the candy bar. So I remembered I was to buy two things and the candy was the second in this case, but it wasn't on the list.

I have been bothered and bewildered but never bored. But I feel my memory is fading faster than I hoped. For the most part it tends to be names, but never ones of people I see or hear from frequently. I have found a trick to remember the names of people we meet. Dorothea recognizes my dilemma and reaches out to introduce herself and that person gives his or her name to her. And Bob's your uncle, as they say.

On the practical side, we've recently learned that increasing the light in the home is helpful and so is sleeping in a dark bedroom. On the home front, we had a rail installed in the upstairs hall at the top of the stairs on the way to the bathroom. The rail will be hinged against the wall to be lowered at night. Skips-to-the-loo at night tend to be more frequent as you age. So, at eighty-four there is a lot of traffic, and I am not one to jump hurdles.

I had a strange memory loss this summer when, with our visitors, we drove up to a lake outside Halifax to see our daughter's cottage, which she and her son Seamus were upgrading. Not only did I forget the way to the cottage, I forgot the cottage itself.

I hadn't been there in more than a year. But I had been there many times and Donna and the others were surprised when I fessed up. I did remember nearby cottages. Go figure!

Before I conclude this column, I'd like to apologize, publicly, to my much-maligned walking cane. It became a godsend on the flight to and from Toronto. Dorothea and I were moved to the front of the lineups at check-in, and we got early security checks and early boarding. I was even offered a wheelchair to get on and off the plane. I told them I wouldn't take a wheelchair unless Dorothea could sit on my lap and have a photograph taken.

In my next column I hope to address the question of privacy rights for those in care. I will try to ensure that my protection of privacy column will not be a downer. I have rounded up people I respect who will help. One friend has practical experience and two have experience with privacy laws. I hope to make it interesting enough for those who read it.

With all that, I am still walking on the sunny side of life, to paraphrase a song of years ago. I hope it continues.

26

My Dancing Days Might Be Coming to an End

Published October 14, 2016

I like attention, but not when I attract the attention of a busload of people.

I was out walking alone recently, when I fell face-forward onto the sidewalk near a bus stop. The driver and a passenger, Paul, hurried off the bus to help. The driver got back to the bus and Paul stayed with me, helped me up, and walked me home.

I was bloody, bowed, and shaky.

Dorothea invited the good Samaritan in to get the story. He stayed for a while, answered the many questions Dorothea had for him, and she drove him to where he was going.

I was bloodied and almost bowed. Very shaken when I was picked up, I can remember feeling uncomfortable on my walk home, but before I could gather my wits about me, I went down.

It's a hell of an experience, knowing you are on your way to a face plant. We are grateful to Paul, and I believe we may stay in contact. He was very sensitive.

A lot of blood spilled. Later in the day, we found blood on the railings up to our back door. My daughter-in-law Carol, a wonderful nurse, hurried over to check me out. She lives across the street. She was thorough, checking eyes, fingers, elbows, and knees. She also checked my nether region to look at my hips. My son, Carol's husband, politely turned his back.

Carol told me to see my doctor and, of course, Frank saw me immediately. He decided to make an appointment at the Falls Clinic, which I had been to eight years ago, before I was diagnosed. Frank mused that the result would not have been as severe if I had fallen on the side of my hip replacement. My face was pretty scary. I looked like I had lost a fight with Cassius Clay.

It was the second time I have come home to Dorothea after falling. The first was while walking a year ago. I had been told when I first got the news that unsteadiness goes with Alzheimer's.

We sent a picture of my mashed face to a young doctor friend in Toronto, the daughter of long-time friends. She is, fortunately, strong-willed, and I love her, so I listen when she tells me a cane is not safe. I now use a weird four-legged cane, but she and Dorothea are pushing for a walker. Hard to see how I'm going to win that one. But it can be tough. I will no longer walk alone, which was a wonderful, pleasant thing for me to do. Thinking time. Walking with someone isn't the same.

I felt I would hide out and stay home for a while but decided to go to my barber, Leroy, and he and other customers got the whole story. One of them recognized me, even with the scars, as the guy who writes the column.

Dorothea oversaw the clipping.

I went back to the gym less than a week later. The scars had healed a little. Owner Dale gave me solo time, carefully watched me, and suggested some changes for the time being. But I got through a round and will be back to my usual two rounds by the time you read this column.

But as Dorothea puts it: My dancing days are over. Maybe.

I had promised a column on the privacy rights for people in care. I have delayed it because soon I will be attending an Alzheimer conference where privacy will be discussed.

27

Privacy Issues Are Acute
for Patients

Published November 5, 2016

Because I know that I will, most likely, have to spend some years in care, I am concerned about my loss of personal privacy. I was sensitized to this issue when I was Nova Scotia's first information and privacy commissioner.

There is a point where people with dementia do not really care about their privacy and cannot do anything to protect it. However, at an earlier stage, when they have all their faculties, they do have a sense of privacy and dignity they've wanted to protect their whole lives. How can these rights to privacy and dignity be protected even when that person can no longer "care" and can't do anything about it?

There are occasional outrageous violations of privacy in nursing homes, such as the posting of pictures of deceased residents in a PEI home within the last year, and other incidents throughout North America. I recognize it is not simple to assure absolute privacy for people in care. There was a time, I am told, that staff in care homes left their phones in their lockers. It's acknowledged that staff now carry cellphones in their pockets, for many good reasons. Many are fathers and mothers who provide their numbers to their childcare agencies. And they may need to call home. I'm okay with that. Of course, cellphones are also cameras. Visitors are advised that if they want to take a photograph of a relative or friend, they must ensure no other patient is in the picture.

I'm told that hospitals, as expected, have privacy policies, which all employees are familiar with and reminded of. My daughter-in-law Carol, a nurse, believes all nurses are aware of the importance of patient privacy but they accept there will be more challenges as technology progresses.

So, I am satisfied care homes and hospitals are aware of the need to protect patients' privacy. There will, of course, be lapses. But I know there are rules and regulations, and that action will be taken if they are offended. I'm told the Department of Health comes into each licensed facility unannounced a minimum of twice a year. If information about a patient is posted in places like the inside of a client's medicine cabinet or bathroom, or if a client's diet is posted on the side of the fridge in the dining room, the home gets cited, and has to explain why it is there and what measure they will take to see it doesn't happen again.

There are also policies and operating procedures when privacy breaches do occur. A good home will advise the competent client or substitute decision-maker as soon as they know a breach has happened and will keep them up to date as the investigation into the situation progresses. Discipline always happens when an employee breaches client privacy. I can live with that.

Even for people with dementia living in their own homes it is important that their family and friends also respect their dignity and privacy within the context of providing care and looking after their safety. As a society we need to pay closer attention to safeguarding the dignity, including privacy rights, of some of our most vulnerable citizens, which includes the growing numbers of older people, whether or not they have dementia.

Human rights commissions, privacy commissions, and other agencies need to pay closer attention to the human rights of the aging population and be more vigilant and proactive in protecting the vulnerable elders who are less able to assert their own rights. It appears that the ethical issues are seriously underfunded.

I recently attended an Alzheimer Society conference in Halifax for those who work in home-care facilities. The turnout was substantial. I was encouraged by the amount of input from those attending.

In my next column, I will score my trip through the maze of dementia. Dorothea will provide her findings. The challenge for me is trying to remember what I forgot.

28

My Friends Don't See a Change, but I Do

Published November 26, 2016

So how am I doing more than four years in?

Let the gods prevail. My eighty-fifth year, coming up next spring, does not bode well, but not bad, nor should I expect it to.

The dawdling days are coming to a close. My friends say they see no change and I know some of them would tell me if I asked. But I do see change and so does Dorothea. I think I have mood swings, but they don't last long. Sometimes, sitting in my comfy chair, melancholy descends. Although I may bathe in it for a while, I don't entertain it for long. As my mother would have said: "Give yourself a shake!"

It is more difficult for me to read if there are any distractions. I compare that to Dorothea's ability to lose herself in a good book. Or perhaps she just tunes me out. I write notes for upcoming columns and can't remember what I wanted to say. Nor can I always read my handwriting. I scribble notes for my columns on a pad near my den chair. By the time I bring it upstairs to my computer, I can't read them. Because I have been using typewriters and computers for more than half a century, penmanship skills are gone.

I avoid complicated newspaper stories; perhaps I can lay that at the feet of the journalist. I was listening recently to CBC Radio's *The Current* when I was told I could "download the podcast." Sure, Anna Maria, I'm right on it. After that I'll get a handle on Bill Morneau's musings from Ottawa.

I can probably be forgiven for a growing frustration since my second face plant. Walking alone was medicinal and that's off the menu now. And that probably increases frustration. To my wife's chagrin I tend to think all quiet times must be filled.

I am forgetting more names I would not normally forget. Not, however, of family and friends. That may come before I go. In an Ian Brown column, he writes that Gord Downie of the Tragically Hip says forgetting names leave holes in his patter. For me, it is frustrating but not embarrassing.

And then there is humour.

I was dressing recently and put on a short-sleeve shirt which had been put away until spring. I didn't notice until Dorothea pointed it out. Putting on my socks is often difficult with gnarled hands. Having donned one recently, I sat looking at my bare foot. Dorothea strolled by and said, "It's the left one." A gale of laughter followed.

I've been thinking of retrograding to using a walker for safer walking and for peace with Dorothea and friends. For me, that's a huge step, so to speak. You can walk safely with it and sit on it occasionally when tired or, God forbid, I feel another fall coming on. There is a vision in my mind of me sitting for a rest on Quinpool with passersby dropping quarters into my lap.

I will accept the walker in the spring. Dorothea's will will prevail. Until then, I am using a single cane with four legs. Next year, both of us will be in our eighties, one looking after the other. We will have to wait to see how it plays out. I promise to accept what my wife proposes. I can predict the future no better than I can remember the past.

Grandson David dropped in one day and asked Nana if Granddad would get better.

In my next column, [the *Chronicle Herald*] obliging, I will write about a wonderful evening Dorothea and I had at a donor thank-you reception. One of the speakers was a medical doctor who has dementia. Another was a brain surgeon who fascinated all of us, particularly me, with his demonstration of two donated brains, one healthy, the other not. The journalist comes out in times like this, and I got a friendly poke from my "guardian" for taking over the session.

Now, a confession. I was not christened "Darce," though I've been called that since before I started school. It is Gerard James Robert Fardy. I seem to remember that St. Gerard Majella was the patron saint of expectant mothers. Really.

I think my wonderful younger sister Mary gave me my name because she couldn't manage Gerard.

2017

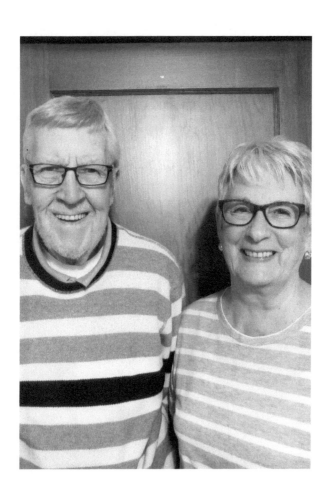

29

Got Dementia? Don't Be Embarrassed

Published January 7, 2017

It just occurred to me that I am more than half the age of Canada, though I wasn't born in Canada. A bare majority of Newfoundlanders voted to join Canada in 1949. I didn't have a vote. I was seventeen. I'm proud that most agree that the island kept its culture.

Before Christmas I was thumbing through *Atlantic Books* magazine to look for books the family might get me for gifts. I chose Ray Guy and Lisa Moore books. When I reached for the book I was then reading, there sat Ray's and Lisa's books looking down on me. Even that doesn't make me fret...just laugh.

Well, here we are...another year. All of the family were here: Sheila, Gabrielle, and Patrick from Toronto; Peter, Carol, Amber, and David from across the street; Donna, Seamus, and Molly, a few blocks away. And all of us in a Christmas mood. This, of course, has been a very special one. They are all aware of their granddad's decline.

We have had them all for Christmas since they were youngsters. Now some of them are borrowing the car. And they all get together so well it's a pleasure to be among them. In my next column I will try to address my mixed emotions during the Christmas season.

And yes, there is always laughter, a good medicine. Recently, Dorothea and I were heading into a store when a woman came by navigating one of those walkers to which I am sentenced in the spring. Dorothea had walked on into the store. The woman, seeing my four-legged cane, admonished me to use a walker. When she went ahead, she stopped to tell Dorothea I would live longer with a walker and added: "I don't know how you would feel about that."

As you might guess I talk a lot. At dinners and drop-ins with people I hadn't seen for a while I retell my funny stories. For Dorothea it could be the umpteenth time she heard it. If only you could hear eyes rolling.

A recent newspaper story was headlined, "What to Get Someone with Dementia." Among the suggestions: magazine subscriptions, automatic medical dispensers, gym membership. I have no idea what an automatic medical dispenser is. I live with mine.

I take ten a pills day, at breakfast, dinner, and bedtime. Dorothea has to keep an eye on the process, as I do after all have memory problems. As a curious old journalist, I suspect some of them may be placebos. I know of no evidence that the pills I take are slowing the creep of dementia.

We often wonder how I would fill my time if I didn't write these columns for the *Chronicle Herald*. I fear I might be sitting in the den reading, particularly in wintertime—reading and napping. The response on the street enervates me. Alzheimer's specialists agree that a wonderful antidote is exercising and socializing, and I can do both at my gym.

And where would we all be without the work of the Nova Scotia Alzheimer Society? I have been able to chat with a number of people affected by the disease, either with it or connected with someone who has it. A friend has someone in his family with dementia. I suggested he contact the Society. He did and was encouraged. I believe he spoke several times to staff.

I want to say I am lucky to be an extrovert, and I recognize that many aren't. I hope that all of those with dementia will share their experience outside the family. It's nothing to be embarrassed about.

And next Christmas? Que sera sera!

30
Sometimes You Just Need to Suck It Up

Published January 28, 2017

It can't be helped. When you are diagnosed with dementia, you are marginalized. No one can help that. It's not intentional but inevitable. And you've just got to "suck it up."

No one's at fault. It's part of Alzheimer's. It's inevitable at times like Christmas. The house is busy, the car is gone from the driveway (driven by a grandchild), gifts are being wrapped. I am no longer in play, as they say. It just happens.

I told the assembled grandchildren that, although I was with Nana when she bought Christmas gifts for them, I'd have no idea what was in the gift as they opened them. We all laugh. To fuel it all, I thanked Donna for the book she gave me. She didn't, Dorothea did. I don't seem able to keep up to speed on the goings-on at home, certainly not at Christmastime. Likely because I'm distracted or I'm a poor listener.

As challenging as some of it was, we had a wonderful time at our annual Boxing Night party. Thirty-six people, most of them friends of Sheila, Peter, and Donna, turned up. Some of them hadn't seen Dorothea and me for some time.

There was lot of food and "fuel," including Manhattans, my favourite drink, which I now seldom enjoy. But I figured that with Donna keeping an eye on me she might use some discretion. It's not my doing. Friend Wayne got me onto them. And now when he and Jo Ann come for dinner, I MUST not let him drink alone. Just not polite.

No one at the party was uneasy with me hanging around. I didn't expect they would be. We had a wonderful visit after Christmas from one of my nephews and his wife. Geoff is the son of my oldest brother, Hugh, and his wife, Kay. His parents have both died. I am the only one of the four Fardy boys, the only one of a family of six children, still kicking—physically, anyway. It was challenging for me to keep a handle on the conversation. And to who was related to who and how.

I've noticed recently that I'm very unsteady when I'm out after dark. I'm never alone. Now there is always someone hanging onto the old guy. My embarrassment quota's gotta be very high in these situations.

Dorothea and I are very encouraged by the emails and letters we receive. A notable one recently was handwritten and came from a gentleman in Englishtown. The man wrote about my columns and has read them all. He was particularly taken by a column he read in November. He said he read it aloud to his wife and then to his daughter and was prompted to write to me. He described the letter as "from one writer to another." He left me with a hint [of] the song "We Rise Again."

I'd like to meet this man.

Later in January, Dorothea and I were interviewed together by a CBC-TV journalist. Stephanie sat us together on our couch and we both answered questions about dementia—living with it, and being married to a guy with it. It is so important to hear from those who "look after" the person with it. It's tougher to tend than Dorothea admits.

Stephanie, from the CBC French section in Halifax, shared it with the English section. A little flashback here. I was waiting for her and her "camera crew" to arrive, and to help if needed. So I watched for the CBC van. Out popped a young woman and she seemed to be alone. I was alert to help. She opened the trunk, grabbed a bag, and came up the front steps, arms full of camera and audio, but the crew was just one person—her.

I was a radio and TV reporter with CBC a "while" ago, and when we went out to cover stories, we had both a cameraman and sound man (yeah, men).

Stephanie worked in both languages and her work appeared on both networks.

Recently, Dorothea and I drove to the Peggys Cove Road area to exchange a gift. It was one of those boutique shops, elegant and small. I went in with Dorothea and noticed the aisles were narrow and the shelves were stacked with fancy expensive stuff. And there I stand unsteady with the damn four-legged cane.

I thought it prudent that I return to the safety of the car. I swear I heard a sigh of relief from the owner when I went to the car.

31
Another Fall Bruises My Head and My Ego

Published February 11, 2017

I t's difficult to tell this story when I must submit it with expletives deleted.

I am not averse to attention, but an incident at the gym took the cake. I took a tumble off the balance board and fell hard to the floor in the midst of a sweating bunch of shocked "gymsters." People reacted quickly and, as luck would have it, one was a nurse. Anita assessed there was no real damage, if you omit that done to my dignity, but the back of my head bled for a while and my lower back aches a little.

Dale, the gym owner, was quick off the mark and with trainer Al came to my aid. The other clients saw I was in good hands and remained a little stunned, I guess. Anita applied pressure to the wound to staunch the blood flow. She then escorted me to my coat and she walked with me to Dorothea, who, after being alerted, was parked outside.

I was able to walk out unaided, though I'm sure my nurse was watching. I had hoped to pull all this off without Dorothea knowing. "Some hopes," as they used to say. Anita explained what she had witnessed. Dorothea is not easily perturbed.

So we went to see our family doctor and Frank suggested I wear a tight ski toque, even to bed, for a few days to protect the wound from bleeding. It was inventive, to say the least, and we laughed a lot when I said nighty-nite. No Facebook for that pic!

It was some time ago that my doctor made appointments for me at the Falls Clinic. When the first appointment approached, I wondered aloud what it was all about. Well, my two dramatic face plants within twelve months, of course. At the clinic, Dorothea and I were questioned together and separately and learned about what would be happening.

In our second session we got down to it. They led me through some very useful exercises to show me how to use my feet, legs, and even posture to improve my balance. The two hours can be pleasantly exhausting, but very helpful. Tracey is assigned to this old guy and puts me through my paces. I'm even subject to instructions to move my bum. What hath God wrought?

An issue arose at the falls clinic when I discovered no one there was aware I wrote regular columns in the *Chronicle Herald* about my progress/regress. I faked outrage.

Every now and then, or even more often, I scramble words. In a letter recently to a man who wrote me, I said I was "glabberfasted" to hear from him. With a smile Dorothea suggested I probably meant "flabbergasted." There's still lots to laugh about.

I've concluded that those who care for people like me have it a lot tougher than the person they watch.

To confuse me even more, I recently read a letter from the president of the CBC on planned improvements to our public broadcaster. He wants "a seamless experience digital sandbox." The CBC, he wrote, will shift priorities from television and radio to digital and mobile services. A space for us all. I figure this must be English, but I'm lost. I was forty years with the CBC. I retired well before this kind of digital stuff. I'll have to check with my pal Bob, a younger CBC retiree, to translate.

Meanwhile, we had a visit from our financial adviser, who is also a family friend. He came to update us. Dorothea handled this stuff for many years, but he was kind enough to include me in the conversation. I was never able to contribute much to these conversations, but he was polite and directed the talk to me for a while. But sometimes I am needed. In a subsequent visit to a bank manager, I was required to sign some documents. I did as directed.

We had a friend visit recently. He hadn't seen us in a year and said he found little if any difference in me since then. That's nice to hear, but we both see gradual regress as we continue. I have encouraged Dorothea to take a break and have agreed to accept any conditions she lays down before she goes away for a week. Those caring for us must get some time off.

32

If I Laugh When the Cane Drops, It Means I'm Okay

Published February 25, 2017

S o how am I doing? A few moderate mood swings. It usually happens when I am sitting alone. I guess I'm a pessimist at rare times. If Dorothea is late coming home—I check my watch and look out the window.

She usually lets me know by text if she is going to be late. If I hear about an accident in the neighbourhood at night I wonder where my family is. It doesn't dominate, but it's there. I guess it's part dementia and part of the winter blues.

A tough time for me is to watch Dorothea shovelling snow to clear off the car as I sit in the den. She also insists on carrying groceries and packages from the car to the back porch. I understand her concern and try not to show my chagrin. We do have someone who clears our snow, but sometimes we have to go out before he comes. I must be driving her crazy. But we can still laugh.

On a visit to the Falls Clinic, I was advised to use a cane in my house as well as outside. I devised a plan for dealing with the cane when it falls on hardwood. In case Dorothea hears it fall, and she hears everything, I laugh out loud to let her know I didn't go down with the cane. And of course, I wander through the house without it sometimes.

I have made some concessions to ease Dorothea's concerns. I won't reach out for the newspapers in the morning if it looks threatening. Our wonderful delivery person makes sure the newspaper's right by the door, but still Dorothea worries. She likely won't be so concerned when winter leaves.

During the winter I joined the "mall-walkers" society. If Dorothea is out and about shopping at the mall, I wander off to join the other walkers. I am a chatterer and I talk to other walkers. If some people are walking around the other way and we meet again a nod has to suffice. It's a place where I can try walking without my ever-present cane…still holding it, but not using it.

And we can still laugh. Recently, I was talking to my friend Rob and asked how his daughter was doing with her basketball. He told me all about it. Less than half an hour later I asked him the same question word for word. Dorothea nudged and we all laughed.

Recently, Yaser, a young physiotherapist from the Falls Clinic, visited us to check out the safety of our house. Yaser made some suggestions to ensure my safety, but things like railings were already in place. We have already made several changes in stairways and the like. He wanted to see how I managed to take showers, and was satisfied we had a handle on it, so to speak. Grab bars are prominent.

Yaser was fascinated at the top-of-the-stairs gizmo that comes down at night when I get to bed. Dorothea and our handyman, Grant, invented it. Yaser also showed me how to put on my trousers safely but demurred when I asked him to demonstrate.

There is a fine line between being cautious and still doing as much as I am able. We have agreed we need to be cautious but not nervous. I don't think I will ever slip into a muddy hole of despair.

I still enjoy life and don't feel as housebound as I thought I would be after two storms in a week. To deal with it we decided to have a "stay-cation." We slept in, made quick meals, and read a lot. It was wonderful.

I am still reading the newspapers and listening to radio during the day and watching television in the evening. Our favourite TV programs are the newsy kind and British dramas. I am now reading *Stalin's Daughter*, the memoir by Svetlana Alliluyeva, the youngest child of the Soviet dictator, Josef Stalin.

The political nonsense going on with our southern neighbours is beyond any understanding. And I have conceded I will never get the hang of Brexit.

33

Life Sentence: I'm Stuck Using a Walker

Published April 1, 2017

I wore makeup and hairspray the other day. Details later.

Recently, I had a dream I was falling down and woke up before I landed. Later that very day I graduated from the wonderful Falls Clinic and Dorothea brought home a list of changes needed in the house: replace my comfy den chair because it rocks, remove carpet from living room, and stay out of the basement.

There are some recommendations I might dispute but likely won't. It's all about losing my control over events. But that, too, is understandable, and I must suck it up. I imagine an octogenarian giving up his comfy den chair. Perhaps they are putting me on. I now use a cane upstairs and downstairs...leaving one at the bottom of the stairs to be greeted by the other one at the top.

Now the big news: I've been sentenced to using a walker. It's inevitable and if Dorothea says I must, I will.

There's levity even in this. My keeper wants me to look "presentable" when I'm out with the "machine." She has a point. Staying neat and tidy is good for morale—mine and hers. She has noted some stuff I wear, including one particular cap, must be shunned.

Back to the Falls Clinic. I encourage everyone who is unsteady or concerned to put their names in. I went on my doctor's intervention and both Dorothea and I have nothing but praise for the entire staff. Tracie was my coach, and she did put up with some tomfoolery. But she had the last word. I'm using a walker. Pride left before (and after) the fall.

Our complete course at the clinic lasted about sixty hours. I'm sure we will be back to say hello. Not everyone at the clinic has dementia. Others have different disabilities. All were treated with respect by the staff.

On my scorecard I find there are times I don't have the intellectual energy to learn or refresh my mind to cope with challenges like recording and storing favourite programming for later viewing. I have done it in the past, of course. Fortunately, Dorothea and I enjoy the same programs.

I've also lost the ability to write legibly. I will jot down notes for a column and fail to read them when I get to my computer.

Now to the makeup I mentioned. I had been asked to do a long video interview to accompany a subsequent major fundraising drive by the Alzheimer Society. I thought the cameraman was kidding when he sent me for makeup and hairspray. I objected and then did what I was told. On the plus side, the makeup artist was a recent immigrant from Lebanon, so we spent the time talking about her country while she made the best of my eighty-four-year-old face and hair.

During the on-camera interview, Dorothea sat behind the cameraman to check for any errors I made or relevant information I didn't mention. Dorothea and I are both featured in the fundraising mailout.

I mentioned my wife's insistence that I tidy myself up when I go out. Recently, we put out clothes for Big Brothers. Looking out in the morning I noticed at the top of the clothes bag was the offensive cap mentioned above. She snuck it out. God only knows what other favourite clothes were on the list. I didn't have my eye on the ball. You'd think I'd have some influence.

I am now in my fifth year with Alzheimer's and can't help wondering what might be next. I'm still in good shape, relatively, but am worried I may find myself in hospital for an emergency and not able to answer questions put to me: What pills do I take? Has this happened before? Or even, Do I know where I am? Will I be able to tell staff I'm in pain?

If this is a worry to me while I'm still fairly competent, how worrisome must it be for those further along in dementia? In my view, the hospital staff should include a patient advocate to pay special attention to those with dementia.

I wear on my wrist an Alzheimer chain which contains contact information. Meanwhile, listening to the radio recently, we are told this is "an amazing time to be aging." Sure!

34

Working on Balance in Both Body and Life

Published April 22, 2017

We took our show on the road recently to speak to nursing students in Amherst by video conference, and to young, eager med students at Dalhousie. Dorothea and I enjoyed it a lot. More later.

We were at Neptune Theatre to watch a play about Newfoundland's decision to join Canada in 1949. Joey Smallwood, the leader of the drive for Confederation, became the first premier. (A reminder: 49 percent of voters wanted Newfoundland to remain a dominion.)

I was likely the only one in the audience who knew Smallwood—and I knew him well. As a reporter, I chased him around a bit and reported from the legislature.

To get to the theatre is a story in itself. Son, Peter, and his wife, Carol, drove Dorothea and me to the theatre. When we stopped in front of the door of the theatre all three emerged and came around to help me out of the car.

Passersby may have expected a celebrity to appear—Trudeau, perhaps! Alas! While Peter went off to park, the two girls linked into me and walked me into the theatre and to our seats. I am well beyond being embarrassed by this stuff. I understand their concern.

Appearing before the Amherst students by video conference, it occurred to me that Dorothea should be part of the Q&As. She sat next to me and answered many of the questions that came from the class of nursing and other medical students. We both enjoyed it, though my wife doesn't bathe in public attention like I do. One sidelight: when I answered a question from someone on the screen, my audience laughed. I was surprised. I discovered that Dorothea was shaking her head to indicate my answer was wrong. We are a good pair on the road.

More recently we sat with a group of young medical students at Dalhousie University. They had questions and we both had some answers. They offered us pizza, which we saw on a nearby table and, when we demurred, the pizza managed to be consumed by the students. They were wonderful. We enjoyed it a lot.

There was genuine interest in dementia and its effects. Our Alzheimer Society organized the session.

We also continue to volunteer at a medical clinic, True North. Strangely, they have had a problem getting blood out of this turnip. Three stabs on both visits...so far. Fortunately, I don't mind needles, and watch while they are stabbing. They are perplexed. I go home with two Band-Aids. Perhaps they'll practise before I am offered up again.

My memory does not appear to be fading dramatically. For some reason I am able remember the middle names of my three brothers, all long gone. Not useful but there you are.

What is useful? Well, some of you may remember I wrote *My Story* for my grandchildren about five years ago. Soon after I finished it I was diagnosed with dementia. Serendipitously it's now a reference book for the columns I write.

I have concluded that, while I spend a lot of time on my balance problems, I'm also concerned with balance in my life. I will be eighty-five in a few weeks, likely not a long time left. I don't want to spend too much of that time on my body balance and forget my life balance...as an old guy who needs to do more during my remaining time to enjoy my life and Dorothea's, beyond the dementia bubble. She agrees.

We are now spending some one-on-one time with Terry, a medical exercise trainer. He provides some guidance for the two of us.

Terry has prepared some exercises. I have been going to Slim's for some time and Terry's recommendations will be used occasionally at the gym. On those days I will have a member of Dale's staff watching over me. That responsibility falls on Leanne, who is about sixty years younger than her charge. She's wonderful. She even enjoys my stories—or fakes it.

But as I say, we can't neglect our life outside the bubble. I will try to spend more time on this issue in my next column if [the *Chronicle Herald*] continues to oblige me.

And a now a tribute to my good friend Jean. She is ninety-five years old and lives alone, goes to parties and, get this, she never uses a cane. Humph! Daughter Brenda and her son-in-law Tom live a short drive from her home. So, all is right with the world.

And now the essential brightener. On a frigid day I found in the closet a scarf I had forgotten...the long kind that wraps around your neck.

I showed it off to Dorothea. Her reaction? I bought it for her when I was in Lima. I can't win.

35

The Bicycle Bell on the Walker Means It's Me

Published May 20, 2017

Free at last, free at last.

The much-maligned walker has arrived, and I have walked the neighbourhood alone. The first time in many months. My daughter-in-law, Carol, a wonderful nurse, walked with me to see to it I handled it properly. Best advice: don't push it, walk with it. Carol also gave me a dandy bell to go with it. If you hear it on my walks, that'd be me.

To cope with this new mode of travel we have adopted a slogan: be cautious, not nervous! Nervousness has a paralyzing quality to it.

For early days, I will tell Dorothea where I am going and stick with that. I can always text her, or she me, if there's a change of course. Dorothea named the machine Willie, to recognize son Peter's wonderful rendition of the Willie Nelson song "On the Road Again" at a mental health fundraiser in Halifax. He even dressed like Willie. I hope Willie will be on the road a lot.

A little pathos. At the supermarket recently we were approached by a woman who wanted to meet us. She told us that both her grandmother and mother died with dementia. She wept. I put my arm around her. I'm encouraged that, having read my columns, people feel I will be a sympathetic listener.

On a less sombre note, a woman emailed me to tell me how to adjust my den rocking chair, which I had been advised by the Falls Clinic to abandon. I will not abandon it, so there.

So how am I doing? I have to struggle more to read complicated newspaper stories like the French election campaign, but radio and TV news presents no problems. My memory is a bit spotty and will get spottier. But I have a plan.

When I was with the CBC, I was invited to attend the military college in Kingston for a year with a bunch of senior military officers and a few other civilians. We spent time at the college and then flew to countries we had been discussing and met with government officials in those countries. We visited countries in Africa, Asia and the Far East, Europe, of course, and South America. My memory is failing, to put it gently, so I dug out the photo albums from those times. With Seamus, my grandson, we went through an album of photographs of a visit we had to Asia.

Back to the present...and the future. I falter when I get tangled in detail. We are taking all this day by day. I'll be eighty-five in a few weeks. That's a big number, although I don't feel old, and Alzheimer's will eventually produce a potent brew. But I'm sure I will remain a garrulous old man. In fact, I don't see myself as an old man. I talk a lot, of course, and that provides Dorothea with many opportunities to ignore me.

The family went to see *Once* at Neptune Theatre. The stage was an Irish tavern, and the audience was invited to go up to the bar and have a beer before the show started. A great musical. It was a wonderful evening with family and, as I sat there, I considered how wonderful life is and how fortunate I am to be able to be fully engaged in living in my fifth year with Alzheimer's.

Recently, Dorothea and I attended an early dementia conference organized by the Alzheimer Society. I assume half of those attending have dementia and the others are their minders. A number of people approached me to talk about the value of my columns.

Sitting in front of me was a man with his mother. He wasn't there out of obligation; he was there because he wanted to be. We discussed Medic Alerts because I have had one for some time and he wants his mother to have one. It was a very enriching conference, with the smiling staff making every effort to ensure everyone was comfortable.

I continue to advise people with dementia that they stay active. As you know, I go to a gym three days a week. Socializing is also promoted and there's lots of that at the gym. I suggest you choose a gym within a short drive of your home. Distance can inhibit regular attendance.

Recently, Dorothea was listening to the radio when I interrupted. That'd be me. She was distracted from the interview, but I told her I would tell her later.

"No," she said. "You'll forget."

36

Hey, Mayor Mike!
Want a Sidewalk Inspector?

Published June 10, 2017

So, we old people have been told there are too many of us. Stats Canada reports there are more of us than of them. Wonder what that means? As columnist Sandra Martin writes, older people "are not shuffling off this mortal coil as quickly as some would like." When you're eighty-five and have Alzheimer's, you may be ready to shuffle. Not me, not yet.

I have been in touch with Sandra and am happy to recommend her book *A Good Death: Making the Most of Our Final Choices*. She makes the point that "not all pain is physical." The future does not bode well for the elderly or infirm. The author notes that, in 1981, on average, Canadians died at seventy-six. In 2006, it was eighty-one; in 2036, 40 percent of us will be living until ninety.

All these survivors will go through several years in ill health. She describes "bored seniors languishing in warehouses with every moment programmed from eating, sleeping, and bathing." An awful prospect.

This information prompts me to encourage our members of the legislature to put aside differences, pocket their slingshots, and take on this "threat" to growing old in peace, for the sake of people like me and our families. Now that the election is over, let's do it. Let's set up a legislative committee, perhaps a committee of the whole. Bring in the experts: physicians who deal with the aging, those who care for the aging, staff of the Alzheimer Society and others.

There's lots of frustration with dementia...angst, even. My sleep is not good. I don't know if I'm having restless sleeps or sleepless rests. The challenge is not to let the frustration take over my life and to avoid slipping into a deep pool of despair. I can't imagine I will, and neither can my friends. Another challenge is to avoid being too self-centred. It sure isn't all about me!

You know the source of my strength? Dorothea, family, and wonderful friends. Writing these columns is a wonderful distraction. I'm glad I thought of it and pleased [the *Chronicle Herald*] obliges.

Well, I'm getting the hang of my walker. I walk the sidewalks in my neighbourhood for exercise and fresh air. So if Mayor Mike wants a sidewalk inspector, I'm his man, for a modest retainer. I did notice that many of the stores on Quinpool Road lack access for my machine. And some of the sidewalks can present a challenge. Willie, my walker, will be happy when we can get out of town.

Meanwhile, I am losing more names, which provokes me to use the four-letter word: "fret." The thought of losing the names of family and good friends bedevils me. I'm not in that "let this chalice pass from me" mode...yet. I'm still content and often happy. But I think from time to time how important it is for me to "die with dignity" and preclude a future where I need to be bathed and fed. I'm not optimistic, but I am hopeful that this eighty-five-year-old body will pack in it before the worst. But not yet! Perhaps it will be "not yet" for a long time. My family will always be part of the discussion.

To end on a brightener, I found on my laptop recently directions to the Arts and Culture Centre in St. John's, NL, of all places. When I clicked on the instructions it started in front of my Halifax home: Down Oak and Connaught and on and on and on. Really. For a guy who started working at the CBC with a manual typewriter and carbon paper it's a huge move to iPhones and Facebook.

Finally, a family story. Grandson Seamus asked his nana if he could borrow the car. I scolded him for not making the request to the head of the house. He replied he did. His nana and I agree it speaks volumes for the way our family is dealing with this matter. No faux pity.

37

Another Fall, This Time with Broken Bones

Published July 15, 2017

I went out for carrots and got home with a broken shoulder. The carrots were needed for a family seal flipper [pie] dinner chez Fardy the next day courtesy of Dorothea's brother Doug, who was visiting from Newfoundland.

I fell hard and did not realize it. Some good Samaritans picked me up and off I went—not knowing a bone was broken. My favourite crossing guard noticed something was wrong and made me sit down, and got a bandage for my knee, which I had not noticed was bleeding, and off I went again.

An x-ray showed a bad shoulder break, which could take months to mend. I'm in a sling facing big challenges. Subsequent x-rays show a broken bone in my back, which will heal itself in time. So writing this column is labour intensive. Only my right hand is useful. There are many pills, and side effects are unpredictable.

Our entire family came for the weekend to cheer us up. We have all agreed Dorothea is becoming exhausted, so she has arranged to spend time with her good friend Sylvia away from all this later in July.

I was really anxious about having personal care. I felt it would be very embarrassing but found, instead, that the personal care worker was so professional and respectful that I need not have worried. Still, being naked in front of a stranger is something one doesn't expect. I can't believe I'm writing this! God has wrought a lot this time, but my wife and I will prevail.

It is never impossible to find humour.

Before I fell, we decided it was time to get a special parking tag for the car. We find it difficult to manoeuvre on foot through parking lots because of my balance problems. My doctor signed on and we hung the tag on our rear-view mirror.

On our way home we stopped at Costco and, as we always do, went looking for a vacant spot. When we finally reached the store, we remembered we had the parking tag. Other customers must have wondered why our laughter was out of control.

When we speak of improvements needed to the health-care system, we are not talking about at the quality of care that is available. The health-care providers are wonderful and there are a goodly number of them in our orbit. We just need better access.

We also immediately sought information and advice from the Alzheimer Society and, as always, they came through with flying colours.

And, believe it or not, we still have room for laughs.

Being of an age when visits to the loo are a big part of the night, calling Dorothea from a deep sleep in the other room can be a challenge.

Friend Wayne MacKay had an idea. He brought us a bell once used in the one-room schoolhouse he attended. It sits by my bed. I ring it when the bladder calls. The wonderful woman, who, I joke, helps me clean house, Joann, gave me a downstairs bell.

38

That Broken Shoulder Wiped Me Out

Published September 8, 2017

I missed the early summer colours. I hope to get mobile for the autumn colours.

Broken bones and dementia form a potent mix, but we have some good news. The broken shoulder has been repaired. Freedom from the sling approaching. We were concerned. For a while, I will use the sling sparingly until my next appointment with physio.

The fall knocked me and Dorothea out of much of our summer. But she got away recently to spend precious time with her wonderful friend Sylvia.

I have always been an early riser, often at work around seven. Now I am wed to the bed, crawling in every chance I get. I have a series of exercises that wipe me out.

Now back from the physical to the mental, i.e., my dementia. Distraction is a wonderful aid. We recently enjoyed a plethora of happy distraction at a birthday party for grandson Seamus's nineteenth. Our friend Glenn and his uncle Peter vied for funniest guy at the party but neither of them grabbed the gold medal, or the bronze.

It brought me a sunny day in the misty fog of dementia. It keeps my fret level low.

When Dorothea went off to spend time with Sylvia, daughter Donna and daughter-in-law Carol, a nurse, moved into the breach.

They are truly wonderful. We would be lost without them. Recovery would have been so difficult. Dorothea would not have left.

They got me out for walks to strengthen my balance, they cooked meals, and Donna stayed overnights. Carol took me to physio and stayed so that she could keep Dorothea informed. There was no indication she needed to be somewhere else. I was given a list of exercises which I do every day. I'm wiped afterward and take to bed.

I can handle only short walks, sometimes no more than ten minutes. This is a guy who enjoyed walks from Connaught to the waterfront. Carol supported me as I staggered on my first walk. I got only as far as the end of our long driveway. It's improving. Both Donna and Carol drop in to take me out. Those wonderful women both have children and are both working. Dorothea returned obviously refreshed.

At home I have ankle weights for exercise when I am sitting around. It will strengthen my legs. You may remember balance is a major issue with dementia, which explains how I broke my shoulder.

On a lighter front, Leroy came in to give me a haircut. Leroy is my wonderful barber, great for an argument.

I missed the early summer colours. I hope to get mobile for the autumn colours.

Writing these columns, I'm reminded of the old saying: "That's enough about me, what do you think of me?"

I am pleased with the response I get from my columns; thank you to the *Chronicle Herald* for running them.

39

A Summer of Friendship and Companions

Published September 23, 2017

How rich we are in friends!

With friends like ours, it isn't difficult for Dorothea and me to keep our minds off dementia.

Christine and Bob [Culbert], our long-time Irish friends, were the first of many to arrive. We've known them long before their grandchildren were born. We went to Ireland twice with them and we took them to wonderful Fogo Island.

In Fogo, we came upon a huge shed. I asked a man sitting on his front steps what the shed was all about. Before he had a chance to reply, a woman came rushing up from church with her rosary beads dangling and suggested she set up a shed party. More than a dozen people showed up and the music started, and the singing started. All in miraculous fast time. Lots of Irish songs. The Culberts were at home.

The four of us drove to Grand Pré, a beautiful Nova Scotia village, to visit with their friends, a wonderful couple who live in Toronto. Stephen is an opera singer. Paul teaches yoga, among other things.

They say an idle mind is the devil's workshop. That would be me. As I struggled into a restaurant, cane in hand, I was met by a woman struggling out with her cane. I confronted her on who has the right of way. I asked her what her age was. She was two years younger than I am. So, I claimed the right to enter before she could leave. It brought laughter from her and a bunch of people. Dorothea later told them she was going to take me home if I didn't behave.

David and Debbie provided a huge surprise. We were expecting Debbie, and then a day or so later, David. When the door opened for David, the family came in with him. They brought the whole family. We were not expecting Christian, Kate, his wonderful fiancée, and his sister, Lexi. They all came in the back door together. Dorothea and I were flabbergasted.

Overflow was billeted at Carol's and Peter's across the street. The visit had been planned for months and we were the only ones who knew nothing about it. If that doesn't shake up my dementia, nothing will. A day or so later, we got a visit from a couple from Yellowknife. Elaine and Peter summer on PEI—they arrived with a huge amount of food, including a blueberry pie made with their own hand-picked berries.

As for my dementia, I know I am forgetting more, or perhaps I am filing it in the wrong memory cell. Who knows? It could be my mind wandering instead of listening carefully.

Meanwhile, I got good news. For the first time in a long while, the arm injured in a fall weeks ago has healed and the arm sling I wore has been abandoned. I now exercise to get my arm back to usefulness. I do exercises three times a day—prescribed by my surgeon and a physio specialist—to help get me get back in shape. The injured arm is improving.

In my next column, if [the *Chronicle Herald*] obliges, I will try to provide a dementia score card on how I am doing.

40

Dementia Is Irreversible, but I am Still Enjoying Life

Published October 14, 2017

S o how am I scoring in my efforts to cope with dementia?
I think there is a noticeable advance in the progress of my disease years in, but not notable...if there is a distinction. Dementia crawls and there is no hope of recovery.

I'm finding it difficult to deal with complicated news stories and TV mysteries. Dorothea has to push the pause button to explain what the hell is going on. For that reason, we record our favourite mysteries.

[*Globe and Mail* health] columnist Andrew Picard tells us that more than half a million Canadians have dementia, and the number is growing. He describes it as frightful. Globally, fifty million have it. He lists ways to stave off dementia: read, write, be physically active, be socially engaged, eat healthy food, and sleep well. An accident halted my visits to the gym, but I will be back, and soon, I hope.

Picard writes that there are few things that aging baby boomers fear more than dementia and losing their dignity. I haven't experienced a loss of dignity, likely because of the way Dorothea and my family and friends treat it. Dementia is not a runaway train. You can still enjoy life.

I have many welcome distractions from my dementia. In a big surprise recently, I learned I was presented with a national award recognizing my contribution to promoting open and accountable government.

When I retired from the CBC, I was invited to become Nova Scotia's first freedom of information commissioner under new freedom of information legislation. I was independent, and although the government was required to provide the resources to allow me to do the job, that requirement was never met. I was paid a small daily rate of pay for days worked.

"Begrudged" is how I would define the government's meagre support. There was no personal support for some time. The office has a desk and chair.

One day, Dorothea came in with a table from home to help furnish the barren room. She stuck her name on it and retrieved it years later when I retired at seventy-five. It was then I established the Right to Know Coalition.

The Grace-Pépin Access to Information Award, an annual national award, came as a huge surprise. It was celebrated at a family/ friends reception organized by the current Nova Scotia commissioner, Catherine Tully. The announcement was made in Ottawa by video link. I was surprised when I got to Catherine's office. Family, friends, former office staff, and some who were government employees in my day were waiting for me.

You're right to conclude that this news has nothing to do with my dementia, or perhaps it does. There are always distractions available to us who live under the veil of the disease. We just have to welcome these distractions and not to be embarrassed.

41

My Friends Have Noticed a Change since I Fell

Published November 25, 2017

I often write about the value of distractions for someone with dementia. Well, the latest took the cake...the birthday cake.

Dorothea joined me as an octogenarian. Family and many friends had a party to honour her, and gathered at cottages near Halifax.

I have mentioned Bob and Christine Culbert, our Irish Toronto friends, in an earlier column. Four of their family came to the party with them. We have known Alison and Andrew since they were youngsters. Alison brought her two children, Maeve, who left her beloved horse for a few days, and Dylan, her younger brother and a buddy of mine since he was knee-high. Andrew brought another Alison. Bob brought "sucky Irish music" and we all sang for hours.

Our Sheila danced alone and with others for hours. Peter sang his Willie Nelson. Donna and daughter-in-law, Carol, made sure we were all nourished...in every way. I could go on, but I might be reprimanded for invading privacy. Other partiers included Tom and David, Susan, Elspeth and another Peter, and Wayne and Jo Ann. Our grandchildren were also there but disappeared to a room with a TV set to escape the adult nonsense.

We were honouring the woman who has gracefully faced the burden of living with and caring for a husband with dementia. The tributes paid to her over those days at the cottage left me unable to pay the homage I planned. I choked—so, instead, I sent the tribute to our friends by email.

I believe emotional hiccups go with dementia.

I was chatting with Donna and Dorothea about what they noticed about my dementia during our cottage stay. I seemed completely confused about who else was staying in our two-storey cottage and appeared confused when the guests came down in the morning.

But it's worse. I am now learning from my friends how they have witnessed my decline since my accident last June.

I have asked Jo Ann and Christine to provide me with their views, which I will share with you in my next column. I was in awful shape after my fall, worse than I imagined. Was I going to survive? Would it all soon end? We have chatted about that event recently.

The story I am preparing for my next column contains more comments from friends from that time in the early days after I fell.

On a lighter side, if there can be one, Dorothea's brother Doug was here when I fell last June while going out to get carrots to cook Newfoundland flipper pie. He was back recently with fresh cod, capelin, and squid from Portugal Cove. No carrots to fetch this time.

Not very long ago, we were surprised when we answered the door and a pied piper in full regalia played his way into the hall, followed by the staff of the Alzheimer Society and Senator Terry Mercer.

As I came downstairs, they were surrounding a bewildered Dorothea. They were there to present Dorothea and me with a philanthropic award for our support of the work of the Society. Exciting morning.

Darce Fardy:
A Life in Photos

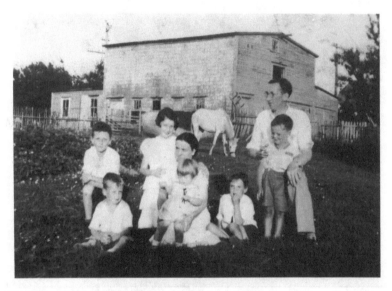

The Fardy family, 1936, in Kelligrews, NL (where the family spent much of the summer). L–R: Hugh, Paul, Marg, Mother (Mary), Mary, Frank, father (Hugh), and Darce.

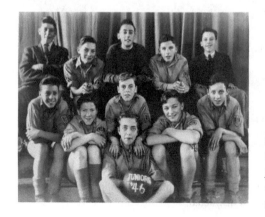

St. Bonaventure's College (St. Bon's) basketball, St. John's, NL, 1946. Darce is upper right—likely team manager.

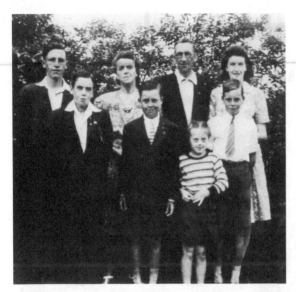

The Fardy family,
c. 1940s, St. John's, NL.
Darce is front and
centre.

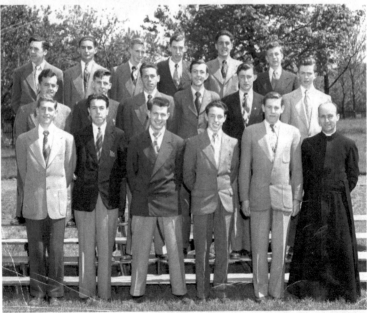

St. Bonaventure's College high school graduation, 1950, St. John's, NL. Darce is in
the back row at far left, obviously distracted.

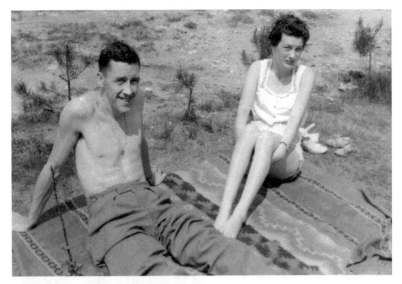

Darce and Dorothea, sunbathing somewhere in Newfoundland, 1957.

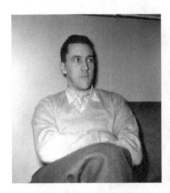

Darce in St. John's, NL, 1959.

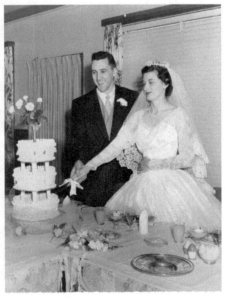

Darce and Dorothea's wedding day, July 2, 1958, St. John's, NL.

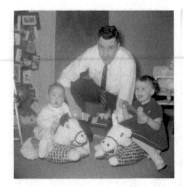

Darce with children Peter and Sheila, Christmas 1962, St. John's, NL.

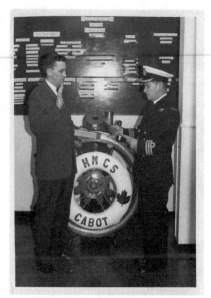

Lieutenant Fardy, Naval Reserve swearing-in, St. John's, NL, 1963.

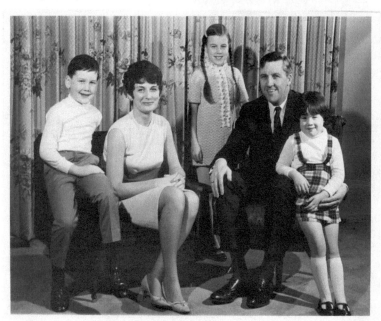

The Fardy family, 1968, St. John's, NL. L–R: Peter, Dorothea, Sheila, Darce, and Donna.

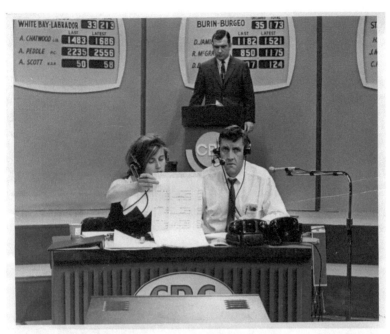

Darce, anchoring the election desk from Newfoundland during the 1968 Federal Election.

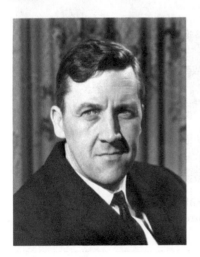

Darce Fardy, 1968.

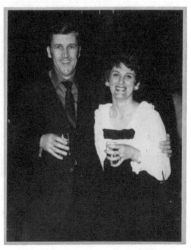

Darce with Dorothea at a reception welcoming Darce to CBC Edmonton, where he did a work exchange, 1969–1970.

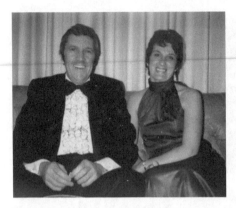 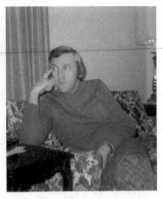

Darce with Dorothea, New Year's Eve 1972, St. John's, NL.

Darce at home in Halifax, NS, 1977.

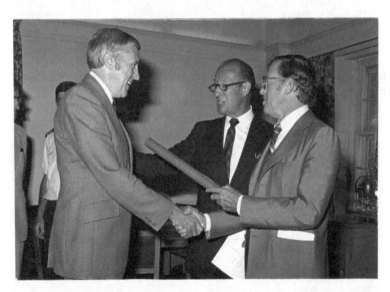

Darce with Minister of National Defence Allan McKinnon, marking the completion of the National Defence College course in Kingston, ON, 1980.

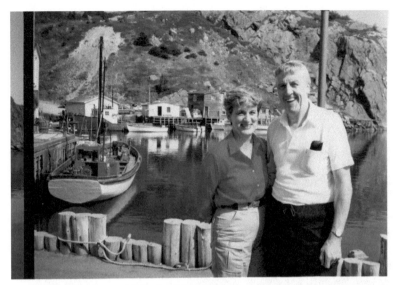

Darce with Dorothea, c. 1980s, Quidi Vidi, NL.

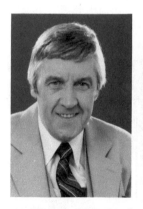

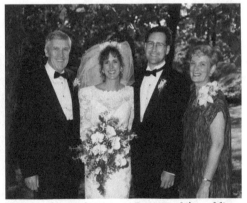

Darce's CBC publicity head-shot from the 1980s while he was head of TV Current Affairs, Toronto, ON.

Darce and Dorothea at son Peter Fardy's wedding to Carol, 1991, Halifax, NS. Darce had just retired from the CBC. L–R: Darce, Carol, Peter, and Dorothea.

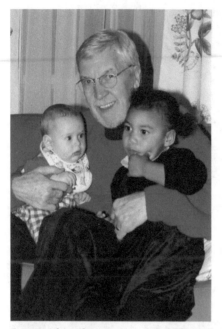

Darce with nephew Seamus, left, and niece
Gabrielle, c. 1998.

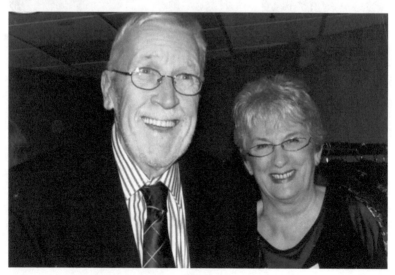

Darce with Dorothea, c. early 2000s, Halifax, NS.

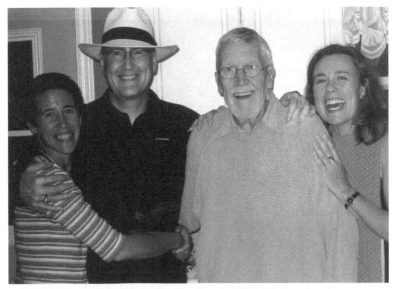

Darce with son, Peter, and daughters, Donna (left) and Sheila, c. mid-2000s, Northport, NS.

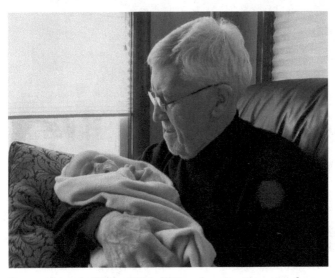

Darce at home in Halifax, NS, in 2004, welcoming a new grandson.

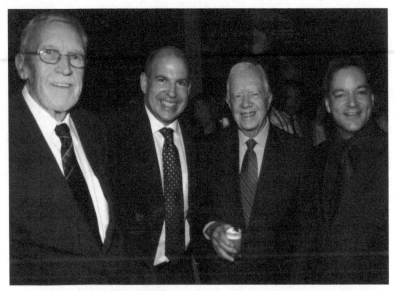

Darce, left, and other Canadian delegates with former US President Jimmy Carter (second from right) at the Freedom of Information conference sponsored by the Carter Institute in Lima, Peru, 2009.

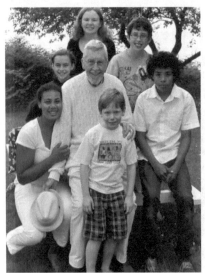

Darce, pictured here with all six grandchildren on his 80th birthday, 2012, Petite Rivière, NS.

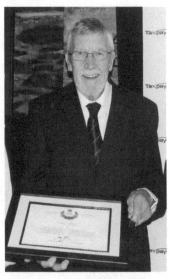

Darce receiving the Queen's Diamond Jubilee Medal, 2012, Halifax, NS.

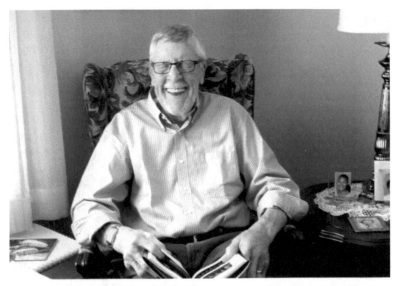

Darce at home c. 2015 in Halifax, NS—finding something funny, as he often did.

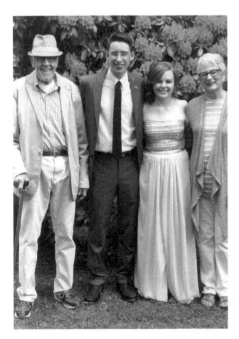

Darce, left, and Dorothea, right, with nephew Seamus and niece Amber celebrating their high school graduation at the Halifax Public Gardens, 2016.

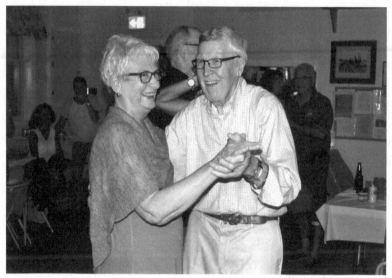

Darce dancing with Dorothea at Peter and Carol's 25th wedding anniversary celebration in Northport, NS, in 2016.

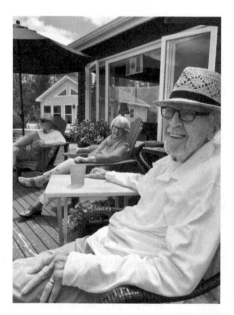

Darce at the family cottage in Northport, NS, with Dorothea and Peter, 2017.

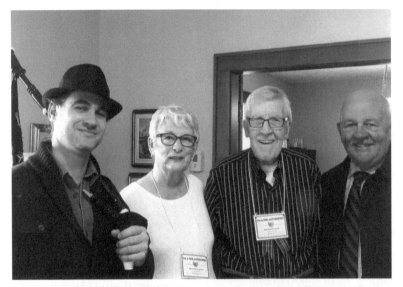

Dorothea and Darce at home, in Halifax, NS, being recognized by the Alzheimer Society on National Philanthropy Day, 2017.

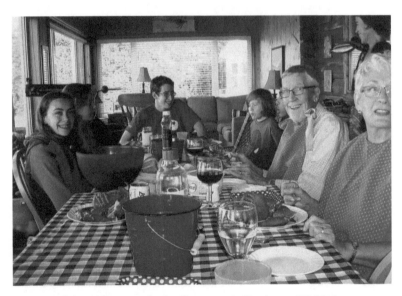

Enjoying a lobster dinner at the family cottage in Northport, NS, 2018.

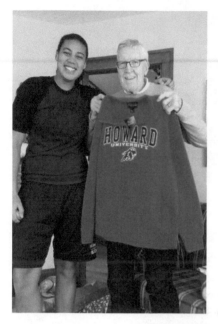

Darce with niece Gabrielle presenting Howard University swag, 2018.

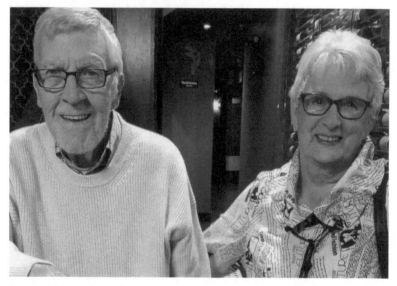

Darce with Dorothea, 2018.

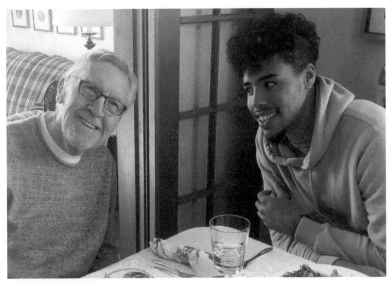

Darce with nephew Patrick at home in Halifax, NS, 2019.

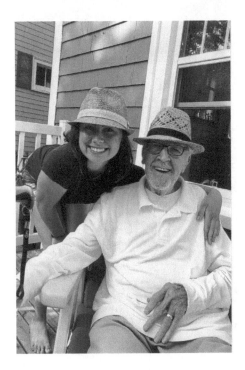

Darce with niece Molly at home in Halifax, NS, 2020.

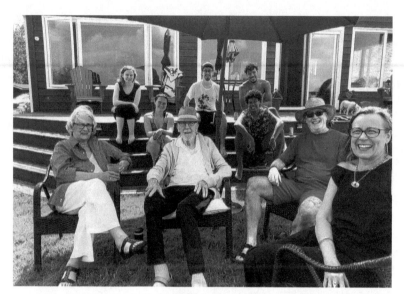

Summer 2021—Darce's last visit to the family cottage in Northport, NS.

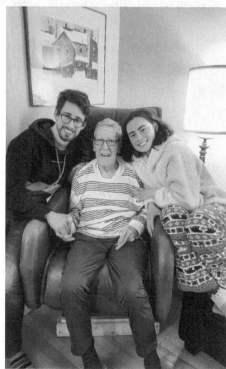

Darce at home in Halifax, NS, with nephew Seamus and niece Molly not long before he died in March 2022.

2018

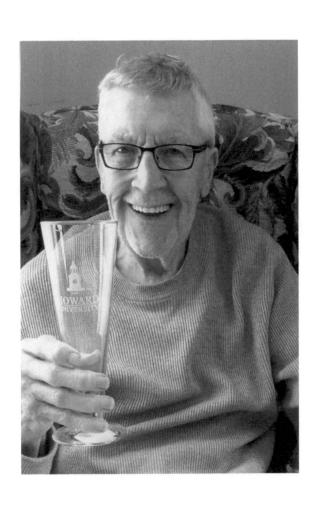

42

Christmas Guests are Patient with My Forgetfulness

Published January 27, 2018

For a guy closing in on eighty-six and having dementia, there's a fine line between pessimism and optimism. And I'm in dead centre. And I hope I can stay that way 'til the end. Pessimism helps no one.

Every day I notice the decline, physically as well as mentally. I am often tired, but not from doing anything. I continue asking my wife, Dorothea, to repeat names for me, often in the same conversation the name was mentioned. That's a patient woman.

Christmas posed a few challenges for me as I tried to remember who gave me gifts and what they were. But having the whole family together for Christmas was a wonderful reward.

Dorothea managed to throw the annual Boxing Day party. Most of those invited are friends of Sheila, Peter, and Donna, but they're friends of ours, too. Most of those there I hadn't seen since the last Boxing Day, but none of them was uncomfortable, and I appreciate that. I remembered many of them. Some provided gentle reminders. Some of them discussed their experience with dementia in their own family.

And I got a lot of hugs.

Recently, Dorothea and I did a video promoting the Alzheimer Society. It has been shown on CTV. One of the scenes had me serving Dorothea a cup of tea. I did it solemnly, not like I usually do, pouring hot water on a tea bag and taking it into the den. Donna thought it funny watching me sweep aside the sheer curtains on the living room window and getting away with it. Not usually done. I don't just put a good face on all this. I'm content knowing that when my dementia demobilizes my mind our family will help their mother through this. Daughter Donna and daughter-in-law, Carol, (a nurse) have been and are providing wonderful support every day. Peter keeps an eye on his mother and is her handyman...he's there when needed. Sheila, our eldest, lives in Toronto. She stays with us while she's here and, in her own vibrant and irrepressible way, takes a load off her mother's shoulders.

On the very day I was diagnosed I stopped driving, relieving the family of that worry.

Some time ago, son, Peter, noticed I was writing a story for my grandchildren. I always wished I knew about my grandparents' lives. He had a number of hard-covered copies printed and each grand-child was given one.

My bet is none has read it yet, but I think they will. The crew that produced the CTV spot that we did for the Alzheimer Society included a shot of that book.

Some time ago, in the early stages, Dorothea and I agreed to go public when asked to sit for an interview with CBC Radio host Anna Maria Tremonti. We think that was a good decision.

I read recently that the average lifespan is eighty-two years. I'll be eighty-six in a few months. For someone with deepening dementia there must be good news there.

43

The Family Discussion about Long-Term Care is Closing In

Published February 28, 2018

S
ix years ago, I wrote *My Story*, a story about my life, to give the grandkids some idea of what it was like in my day. I read it again recently and aced it. I remembered everything.

Dorothea and I have now volunteered for another project. Home-based older adults and their care team...with a monster title: "Caring Near and Far: A Multi-Province Investigation of Remote Monitoring Technologies Connecting Community-Based Older Adults and their Care Team."

It's a project of Dalhousie University. It took a few hours for a member of the investigative team to explain it to us. We are told this study will evaluate whether remote monitoring of homes to allow those in care to be in their homes would be efficient. Sensors would be placed in the home and monitors would be installed to track unsafe behaviours of older adults...and to relieve family or friends. It would show if the person had taken her/his medicines or, for instance, opened the fridge door that day.

We have agreed to support this plan.

I think it is agreed doctors should advise dementia patients that they should not drive. One doctor agrees it represents a loss of autonomy, a loss of self. Another expert is astounded that people see no connection between driving and dementia. You can't drive anymore, as dementia delays your reaction time. Not driving may be a loss of self but it's not worth the risk, in my view. I gave it up and it is a damn nuisance. But I considered issues like kids on bicycles driving by your car. Limiting your driving to short trips is not enough. We need a public health campaign discussing the issue. Physicians should prepare dementia patients, because giving up driving presents a tremendous emotional impact. The afflicted have to reconsider what were once regular mundane tasks, like getting groceries and visiting friends. Driving is indeed a ticket to freedom.

Otherwise, how am I doing? I read *Maclean's* and other magazines regularly. I have found myself rereading an article I had already read. I was into the story when I realized I had already read it. Same with *Halifax* magazine. Not encouraging, but I continue to read.

I think I have lived too long. The last four years have brought on arthritis as well as advanced dementia. My parents didn't live that long, and I don't remember them dealing with the problems I am.

My arthritic fingers knocked over a cup of tea in the den. We concluded that the mishap caused more of a mess than necessary as Dorothea and Carol were on their knees cleaning up.

Proof positive of my memory loss came when I forgot my lotto numbers.

I guess my regress can be noticed in my columns, which [the *Chronicle Herald*] has been so kind as to accept. Sometime I may settle in and reread. The decline may be obvious.

Eventually, perhaps sooner than later, the family will gather to discuss my going into care. I am determined to do that for Dorothea's sake and to ease pressure on the family. And I will not expect daily visits, especially if it comes to me not recognizing them.

I am encouraged by people contacting me...often to tell me about their family's experiences.

I'm still on Facebook and text daily. It's a good distraction.

44

Frustrated, but Still Optimistic

Published March 14, 2018

In my last column I inadvertently led readers astray with what appeared to be a prediction that I would soon be placed in care. I feel I am no closer to that than when I was diagnosed years ago. I regret having left that impression. Some concerned friends contacted me.

Pessimism or frustration? There is a difference. I am frustrated (there must be a stronger word than that to use) but I remain optimistic.

There was a song years ago advising us to "dream when you're feeling blue, dream, that's the thing to do." I've done that in spades. It goes with the territory. I've started having nightmares, horrible interruptions of the night's sleep. A few times I would wake from one and then pick it up again with the same nightmare. Figure that out. I guess it's all part of the dementia experience.

I now have a tablet, a cellphone, and a laptop computer. Getting a handle on the new stuff is a challenge, which Dorothea and the family help me meet. A while ago I gave Seamus, my grandson, my old portable typewriter, carbon paper and all.

Social contact is so important. John Lewis, a wonderful old friend, introduced Dorothea and me sixty-three years ago. They met at Memorial University in St. John's. We are still in contact.

He retired in St. John's after years practising medicine in Africa. He is a Rhodes Scholar (I may be a Rhodes Scholar, for all I know).

John defines his issue as old-age memory loss. He doesn't spend much time on the new ways of emails or texting or reading online. When he was giving me information on the phone about his condition, I asked him to send me the information on email.

I heard him ask his wife if they have email. That's John.

As an aside...I remember the places we are going to but don't remember how to get there.

And I discovered a memory jogger: photo albums. We have a dozen or more of them. They are now old-fashioned, but they are great reminders of years past. I do have to ask Dorothea who's who and what was the occasion the photos reflect.

In the new texting age we live in, I have to be careful not to text to the wrong person. But texting is a wonderful way to stay in contact with family and friends. And I don't have to drag myself out of my comfy den chair.

Dorothea and I are still doing well. My family has no need for worry. The end of winter will provide a new spring in my step. By the time this column goes to print I hope to be back at my gym for the first time since I fell, broke my shoulder, and damaged my back ten months ago. Dale has spoken to my physiotherapist, Janice. I'll build up my strength, starting slowly.

On a recent visit with our friends Gwen and Brian I was surprised to see them shocked by my unsteady gait.

A cousin of Dorothea visited us from Newfoundland. It was fun to listen to them talking about their early days before I came on the scene. She, too, was taking a short break from tending to her husband, whose health issues are much more serious than mine. Those women are strong.

The only bad news is that I don't get all of [Bruce] MacKinnon's cartoons in [the *Chronicle Herald*].

45
Meeting the Most Interesting People

Published March 29, 2018

We have a mystery in this house. I do nothing and am always tired, wiped out even. You can guess who does all the work.

I just finished reading *The Leisure Seeker*, a novel about a couple in their eighties, the husband with severe dementia and his wife with an incurable health problem. The husband more or less goes along for the drive—a long trip along the famous Route 66 in the US. Despite the objections of family, they decide to take to the road in their RV. He would drive because she couldn't, and she would tell him how to get there. They drove for days. She often asks, "Don't you know how to get there?" Sometimes he pretends he does. She is just not convinced "all the memories he has floating in his head are lost."

That book, as well as a book of poetry, were offered to us by a woman we had never met who bought them back from Florida. We will call Marg to come to retrieve the books and have a cup of tea, as we'd like to see her again.

The Leisure Seeker was a tough read for me, poignant but funny, and I soldiered on to finish it.

I also read a story on "deterioration of thinking ability and memory and navigating the stages of dementia." I don't know my stage. Not all of the advice provided to those with dementia fits in my case. Perhaps that's because I have a partner in Dorothea.

I don't know what visiting friends observe, but they are never uncomfortable.

You may remember in earlier columns about drug-testing clinical trials I volunteered for. I experienced wild nightmares. When the offending pills were dropped, the dreams disappeared, but I lost my appetite. So there.

Many Canadians will know who Jann Arden is, a funny Canadian comedian who frolics on television with the likes of Rick Mercer. In a new book, *Pathos and Humour: Feeding my Mother* [sic; the title is *Feeding My Mother: Comfort and Laughter in the Kitchen as a Daughter Lives with her Mom's Memory Loss*], she writes about caring for her mother while continuing her career. Her mother, who lives next door, has flows and ebbs. A wonderful read, but a tough one for someone with dementia.

Recently, I hung around with ninety-four-year-old Jean, who's still plenty sharp. She wanted to meet me. I concluded she wanted to show off how sprightly she is. Donna and Dorothea howled when she bounced out of a chair while I was struggling to stand up. She is lucid and content and speaks lovingly of her late husband.

Dorothea and I are meeting the most interesting people since I went public with my dementia. And life goes on and I enjoy most of it.

46

Return to the Gym Is about More than Exercise— It's Essential

Published April 11, 2018

I t's comforting to know that studies continue on the mystery of dementia.

I have read that the brain tissue lab at Dalhousie University, led by Dr. Sultan Darvesh, has concluded that there's hope for a cure for Alzheimer's or, at least, that one in three cases may be preventable. This comforts me. Dementia is something I hope my family will be spared.

I remember arranging to donate my brain when I am done with it. But there's a caution: I didn't do well in school.

I have wonderful news. I am back at the gym after an eight-month hiatus when I fell and broke my left shoulder. For me, the gym is much more than exercise; it's mixing with other people I would not have met otherwise. But the exercise is essential. Dale was happy to have me back and paid special attention to me while Dorothea sat at the front desk keeping an eye on me.

And then came Dayna, who gives me personal attention. I know she loves me, but what can I do? I still appreciate her patience. Dorothea is watching us even closer. But Dayna doesn't take it easy with me, so as a result I am too tired to flirt. When she delivers me to Dorothea, I'm taken home to rest. Dayna is a lawyer but decided to do something useful like helping an old, demented guy get on with his life.

I have been asked how I can stay in a good mood with that dastardly disease affecting my life. I have no answer to that. Meanwhile I am scrambling to try to remember the names of fellow "gymsters" who are still my friends.

Here's another sign of dementia. I could be in the kitchen when I think I should remind Dorothea we are short of jam or peanut butter or whatever. When I walk into the den to tell her, I forget what it is we need. Dorothea remains bemused.

Staring at me as I sit in the den is a yellow book: *The Newfoundland Dictionary of the English Language* [*sic*: *Dictionary of Newfoundland English*]. My mother used to say I was lazy as a Mahone soldier and an omadhaun. You can guess what that meant. I'll teach you more "Newfoundlandese" in subsequent columns.

I don't want to brag about it, but Newfoundlanders seem to avoid taking stuff too seriously. You may know that we were very concerned about letting our rich-in-lore island join the rest of you. Cape Breton looked promising though.

47

Movies and Memories—and Lots to Look Forward To

Published May 11, 2018

Y ou may remember in an earlier column I wrote about a book I had read—*Leisure Seeker*—which told a story of a woman with advanced cancer persuading her husband with advanced dementia to go for a long drive in their RV without telling the family. With the husband driving.

A movie followed and Dorothea and I wondered if we could sit through two hours of this disturbing drama. We dilly-dallied. Well, we did watch it. At times, the husband was quite unaware he was upsetting his wife and acted irrationally, even to the extent of becoming aggressive with his wife.

I found myself quite emotional and these were times I would reach over and hold Dorothea's hand in an attempt to assure her that wouldn't happen to us. We were glad we watched the film, but it was tough on me and perhaps on her. It was not discussed much afterward.

Going to the gym may not extend my lifespan but it makes it easier for me as I try to stay mobile. I found out I have been there seven hundred times over the years. My friend Wayne boasts he has been to the gym a thousand times. I have to say I appear to be in better shape.

Back home, my behaviour still presents occasions for laughter. Recently, I asked Dorothea on three occasions in one day for the name of the book and movie mentioned above.

As I write this, we are having a tough spring. Summer is close. A blessing for a housebound guy who is in no shape to cope with slippery sidewalks.

Soon Dorothea and I will be flying to Toronto to join the rest of the family going to see *Come from Away*, a Broadway musical created to honour the people of Gander, NL, who housed hundreds of airline passengers turned back from New York when a plane hit the Twin Towers in New York City. The trip to see the musical was Peter's Christmas gift to all of us. We will be staying with wonderful friends in Toronto, the Culberts. I trust they know we are coming.

I will soon be eighty-six. Only one other of us in the eight-member Fardy family of Mullock Street, St. John's, lived to be that age, and her last years were very, very tough.

For now I offer another word from the *Newfoundland Dictionary of the English Language*: "summer kitchen."

The back room was used to make pickles and jams and the like at a time when many mothers did that. Others had stoves for the use of those who spent the summers in Kelligrews, like the Fardy family.

For a while I fell in love with Elsie Tilley, who lived there all year. I also ran into trouble as the young Fardy boy.

I used to listen for the train by putting my ear to the track. When I heard it, I would cross the tracks and wait. As it puffed away, I jumped on the steps to one of the passenger cars and jumped off as it picked up steam. This required running along with the moving train, hanging on for the thrill.

Another Tilley turned me in to my mother.

48

Forgetting is a Central Fact of Life for Me

Published July 12, 2018

Pleasant diversions are a wonderful antidote for dementia. I had them in spades recently.

Son, Peter, and wife, Carol, invited Dorothea, daughter Donna, and me to a no-expense flight to Toronto and tickets to see *Come from Away*, that wonderful stage show recognizing the hospitality that people of Gander, NL, provided to airline passengers unable to fly into New York after the 9-11 terrorist attack in 2001. Daughter Sheila, who lives in Toronto, joined us.

While in Toronto, we spent time with wonderful long-time Irish friends Bob and Christine and their family and grandchildren, including my buddy Dylan, thirteen. His sister Maeve was there as well.

I became a little cranky at the airport on our way to Toronto. Carol insisted I navigate the airport in a wheelchair. I sulked. Didn't need it. What if someone I knew saw me and scoffed?

But get this: we were the first to board and got lots of smiles from airline staff.

Recently, I watched a movie, *Away from Her*, starring the wonderful Newfoundland actor Gordon Pinsent. Pinsent's character's wife was in care and believed that a male patient was her husband.

The thought of forgetting that Dorothea is my wife makes me shudder. I'll drown in a wave of depression. And I want to die before she does. That's the least I can ask for.

How normal is forgetting? "I forget" is one of my often-used phrases. Of course, people use it, but just as an idle comment. For me, though, it's a central fact of life.

I've read somewhere—of course I forget where—that scientists are working on a cure for dementia, or at least on ways to avoid it. If they are looking for a volunteer, that would be me.

For all that, spring has sprung and summer is nigh. It's putting a bounce in my step and wonderful diversions in my days.

I have lots of spare time and try to use it wisely. So how am I doing in that department? Fortunately, I enjoy books, magazines, and newspapers, on- and offline. We have subscriptions to five magazines. I read [the *Chronicle Herald*] and others online.

I have just read *Dispatches from the Front*, the story of Matthew Halton, a famous Canadian war correspondent during the Second World War. It's a wonderful read written by his son David, a CBC correspondent himself. I am also reading *Newfoundland in the North Atlantic World* by David [*sic*: Peter] Neary, and *The Long Way Home* by John DeMont, who writes in [the *Chronicle Herald*].

I also read the news a few times a day on my tablet. Dorothea is a wonderful reader and remembers more than I do.

I also have weird things happening. Whenever we are watching shows on television, I invariably think I have seen it before. Dorothea assures me I haven't. I never know how it is going to end. Maybe some expert can explain what is going on in my muddled mind.

Meanwhile, I know the clock is ticking and my mind will continue to betray me. Without Dorothea I would be depressed twenty-four hours a day.

49

Family and Celebrations Create Pleasant Diversions

Published August 20, 2018

S oon after I was diagnosed five years ago, I knew that my dementia would lay a heavy burden on my wife.

Dorothea was sensible and recognized this and decided she needed a break from the handsome guy she married sixty years ago. So she left with book in hand and spend a few nights at Peter and Carol's cottage. While there, she met a friend she hadn't seen in a while. When she returned, you could see her face more relaxed. I wept when I noticed.

Daughter Donna moved in with me and saw to it that I was fed. Daughter-in-law, Carol, dropped in throughout the day and took me to my favourite haunt, the waterfront market, where I used to hang out every Saturday in the old days. We sat in the sun and enjoyed the harbour. I am blessed with a wonderful family.

Another pleasant diversion for this old granddad was Molly's graduation from high school. Before the ceremony, the young adults gathered at the park on a gorgeous day in their fancy dresses. The young men, including Tony, Molly's friend, wore tuxedos. I hadn't seen Tony without a peaked cap on backwards. He didn't look as comfortable in his finery as the girls did. There were four hundred graduates. They went on stage alphabetically to get their awards. Dorothea and I saw it through to the end.

I also went to David's graduation at Churchill Academy. I sat with Carol, who wept when she was awarded recognition for her service to the academy. As expected, Carol said there were other worthy parents. I held her hand.

On another front, we had a visit from Dorothea's brother Doug Neary and his daughter, Karen, a wonderful young woman. As expected, but not required, he brought fresh fish from Newfoundland waters off Portugal Cove. It was enough to feed the whole family and Wayne, who let us know he'd like fish even though he was a farm boy.

To add to our pleasure, we had a visit from Elaine and Peter, our Yellowknife friends. Lots of wonderful diversions for an old guy with dementia. I still enjoy the gym and the friendships there.

50

I Try to Keep My Questions to a Minimum

Published September 18, 2018

R eaders of my earlier columns commented on my good fortune in having readers react to my writing. I am grateful.

I am also delighted to have visitors. Our godson and his wife, Kate, newly married, came from Toronto to visit us for the better part of a week. Christian and Kate came to see us because we couldn't get to their wedding because of my condition. They came with us to Northport to Peter and Carol's cottage for a lobster party for seventeen people.

The party celebrated the birthdays of grandchildren Patrick and Molly. Patrick's mom, Sheila, came from Toronto for the party. Daughter-in-law, Carol, prepared the cottage for the huge party. Donna, Molly's mom, made salads and birthday cake at another cottage while we picked up the lobsters en route.

The whole family was delighted to see Christian and Kate again.

Two of the family missed the whole shebang. Peter was out of town and Gabrielle had started university in Ottawa. We stayed overnight, and on the way home we stopped in for cookies and coffee with our friends Linda and Owen. Then we spent the afternoon on the beach.

On the way home we stopped at Masstown for fish and chips. Christian did all the driving to relieve Dorothea.

The young couple cooked meals and cleared up. They recognized I had difficulty getting around and were at my side throughout their visit to ensure I was secure. I got a lot of hugs from Kate.

Yet I still forget some names and ask Dorothea questions she has already answered.

We watch a lot of mysteries on television. She follows them and leaves me behind. I try to keep my questions to a minimum. I must say, I feel sorry for those with dementia who may not have the family support I have.

I met a gentleman with advanced dementia a while ago and asked him if he had children. He replied he didn't know. I am grateful that hasn't been my experience.

51

Pessimism Is Sometimes Hard to Avoid

Published October 28, 2018

About ten years ago my son, Peter, suggested that I write the story of my interesting journalism career.

As it was going to print, I was told I had dementia. It was noted in the last pages of the book. And there I was with an uncertain future for me and Dorothea and my wonderful family.

If my dementia is not showing improvement, then it must be deteriorating. But it doesn't feel like that. I'm still alert and curious. I just finished reading *Dispatches from the Front* by David Halton, and am reading Peter Neary's book on Newfoundland's reluctance to let Canada join us. I have no difficulty with words, and Dorothea will attest to that.

There have been discussions about advance directives for people with dementia, but I'm not ready yet. As it stands now, the law requires that you have to be able to consent closer to death, so the only choice I have is to wait and hope.

Things could always be worse.

One man I read about was diagnosed at forty-one. Memory loss starts gradually, but I don't feel I will live long enough to experience the worst of it. I don't want the family to see me as a depressed old man. Old, yes; depressed, no. I have such richness with Dorothea and my family.

I read somewhere that 24 percent of boys get dementia and 35 percent of girls, though there is no explanation of why. Physical activity is stressed. I was aware of that and complied by going back to the gym. There's no need to be embarrassed if others at the gym notice. My columns like this one have already given me away.

I often wonder if, in an advanced state of dementia, whether I will feel grief when others are grieving, happiness when others are happy, sympathy or empathy when appropriate.

Friends often tell me that memory fades as one gets older. That may be so. I am old, eighty-six and counting. How long will I live? Pessimism is sometimes hard to avoid. I'm not walking on the sunny side of the street, but overall, things are not bad.

The *New Yorker* ran a story about a family with a parent with dementia who tried to make his surroundings, wherever he was, look like home. I don't need that. Personally, I am not depressed, for obvious reasons. I have a wonderful family and faithful friends who visit often. In some sense I am fortunate to be a news junkie, thanks to my many years as a journalist. One might not expect a person with my disease to follow the complexities of what is going on, from Brett Kavanaugh to Justin Trudeau. I eat up politics, newscasts, and mysteries.

Meanwhile, Dorothea and I have agreed to join a study by phone of dementia, titled "Exercise as a Strategy for Dementia." The organizer had read some of my columns and got my contact info from the local Alzheimer Society.

So, there we are. It's a weird disease to cope with. I hope to die in clear weather and not in a fog of despair.

52

Living with Dementia is Made Easier by Visits from Friends

Published December 3, 2018

I think I am doing fairly well as far as advancing dementia is concerned. I think Dorothea agrees. I know she is always on alert, but we can still enjoy ourselves.

I relieved her of one substantial worry when I voluntarily decided to stop driving. I read recently that one of the issues relevant to dementia is for the partner of the person with dementia to persuade the other to stop driving. On the other hand, I am probably a bit of a nuisance in that when Dorothea gets into the car, I jump in beside her. She is pleasant about it.

The other day on my iPad I was offered all the information I need to know about dementia. I skipped over that. I am trying to find out why I am so exhausted much of the time. Is it a symptom of dementia or am I just plain lazy? Dorothea considered it very briefly and came down on the side of laziness, if not sloth.

On the gruesome side, I hope to die before Dorothea. She can handle that, but I would diminish without her. I have often thought how I would manage without Dorothea if she died before me. I don't think I could. She is strong.

On the brighter side is our good fortune in having friends visit.

Debbie is a long-time friend of Dorothea and I love her. Her husband, David, is a Toronto lawyer with a handyman's streak. They are the parents of Christian, who visited us earlier with his new bride, Kate. They took pride of place in an earlier column and won our hearts.

Debbie wanted to visit to learn how to bake a Christmas cake, not to see me. Hard to believe. Dorothea bakes about a dozen Christmas fruitcakes this time every year for family and friends.

David used his handyman skills and fixed things that needed to be fixing, such as the lock on the shed door, the handle on the fridge door, and the alarm system. Although I grew up with three brothers, none of us were handy. In Newfoundland, handy also means nearby, so I guess we were.

So, there we are. No cure in sight and none expected. But lots of support from family and friends.

53

Family Helps Me Deal with the Frustrations of Dementia

Published December 23, 2018

Frustration. It's a long word with many consequences. There's no pain with frustration, but that's the only kind thing I can say about it. Frustration is watching Dorothea clear the snow off the car in the driveway. In fact, frustration ramps up when I see her doing so many things I used to do. She struggles bringing the groceries from the car into the kitchen. She is concerned I will fall while I'm helping.

Dorothea muses, aloud, that I was never much help around the house but now I am down to zero. I am often in the way, I expect, but Dorothea doesn't say that.

Because dementia lends itself to unsteadiness or even falls, she is super-conscious of the need for care. So, while she looks after everything, I sit in my comfortable den chair feeling a trifle guilty. Not so comfortable when I watch what Dorothea does every day. She would claim I don't look all that uncomfortable watching her work.

That's enough of that. We had a happy distraction when Dorothea's brother Doug Neary arrived from Portugal Cove outside St. John's and, as expected, he brought along enough fresh cod, capelin, and squid to feed the family and, of course, Wayne and Jo Ann. And he does the cooking.

I always enjoy Dorothea's conversations with her brother about growing up in that village. While visiting Newfoundland recently, Donna persuaded her uncle Doug to get her into Nana's house, now occupied by another family. He did it for Donna, of course.

Doug was also a great help for his sister as she struggles to get me safely into the car. Fortunately, I am entirely unembarrassed being helped into the car and up the steps, and Doug was quite comfortable doing so. As an aside, daughter-in-law, Carol, showed me how to get in the car. Bum first, before the rest of me.

I would like to take advantage of this column to pay tribute to my friend Dayna, who tends to me at the gym and is aware of my balance problems. She has read about dementia and the perils of falling and is assigned to putting me through my paces while keeping me on my feet. I often notice her standing behind me when I am working out. She has her arms stretched to be ready for the worst. And the worst could happen. God help her if I fall and take her with me. Dayna may be able to get up, but not me—and I'm on top. Owner Dale to the rescue if that happened.

2019

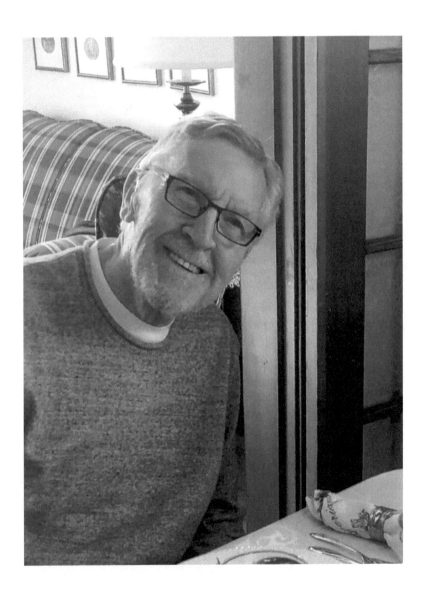

54

Thoughts and Talk of Dementia Are Put Aside for the Holiday

Published January 27, 2019

Well, I found the temporary cure for the dementia doldrums: Christmas.

The whole family, including our six grandchildren, sat around our dining room table to have Christmas dinner together. Thoughts and talk of dementia were put aside for the celebration. In fact, it was pushed aside and buried while we got on with life with our wonderful family. Dorothea and I were on cloud ten with a full table. But it was a close call. Before Sheila and her two, Gabrielle and Patrick, left for Halifax, a fire broke out in their home. We thought our celebration would have to be cancelled. But with the kindness of her friends, some good luck, and Sheila's strength of character, they were able to make it for Christmas.

So the cousins had a wonderful time together. Gabrielle and Patrick Emilien, Seamus and Molly MacInnes, Amber and David Fardy. They found the adults' conversation boring and fled to the den where they played games I couldn't understand.

January is Alzheimer's month. It's a fine refuge for those disturbed by the disease. In early days, Dorothea and I gave our time to the Society with public speaking and speaking to young medical students about life with the disease. They showed a terrific interest.

Perhaps someone in their families experienced the disease. My advice to those who have dementia is to contact the Alzheimer

Society and meet the staff and volunteers. There are more than half a million Canadians with this disease, and there are twenty-five thousand new cases every year.

When I decided to write about my experience, I was pleased [the *Chronicle Herald*] decided to carry the columns.

My friend Wayne MacKay, a notorious hoarder, to his wife Jo Ann's chagrin, saved my columns from the start, more than five years ago, and put them in an envelope. Dorothea saved them as well, of course, and sends copies of them to our friends across the country. But Wayne's recent delivery of them made it easier for Dorothea and me to reread them.

With the *Herald*'s support I will continue them for as long as the paper runs them.

55

I'm Certainly Not Going to Pack It In

Published February 11, 2019

My faculties with respect to dementia, I've read, are being tossed around. Losses of memory, judgment and reasoning, communication, mood and behaviour, and altered visual perception is the result. It sounds like a throw-in-the-towel suggestion, but I am not prepared to adopt that.

Conclusion: I'm certainly not going to pack it in.

I am reluctant to take issue with a conclusion reached by Dr. Ken Rockwood and Dalhousie medical student Lindsay Wallace, who see frailty as a key dementia risk.

"Frail" is a word I haven't heard for a long time, but it is one of those words that sounds like what it means. Dr. Rockwood was available to Dorothea and me when I was first diagnosed. He provided comfort to both of us.

I have to say that before I was diagnosed I was very active, walking for miles from my home on Connaught Avenue to the waterfront market and home again.

After my diagnosis, I began to use a walker outside and a cane when I am home. I grasp both rails when I walk up and down stairs. I fell once outside and damaged my left arm, which still plagues me. However, I eat well, exercise at a gym, and enjoy myself. I never drank much liquor, though I use visits with Wayne McKay to join him with a Manhattan. So there. You['ve] got to have some fun. With respect, that doesn't add up to frailty.

Dr. Rockwood writes that about seventeen thousand Nova Scotians have dementia. That number is expected to double over the next twenty years or so. I have lots of company. Ms. Wallace advises that if we are old, there is a pack of health issues that go with dementia. I'm eighty-six, but as I have said in earlier columns, I read books and newsmagazines and stay alert on what's happening in the world. And I'm a curious kind of guy. Perhaps my journalism career helps. I'm not vegetating. Dorothea wouldn't allow that.

I've read that, along with memory loss goes judgment, reasoning, communicating (what I'm doing with this column), mood, and behaviour. I'm not moody. Dorothea, my mainstay, may sometimes wish for silence from me, but she knows that's a lot to ask.

56

Worry Comes with Dementia

Published March 3, 2019

"Worry" is the word of the month for me...
Worry about Dorothea and whether she can sustain keeping an eye on me and my dementia.

I'm told by the experts that what I can expect beyond memory loss is changes in judgment, reasoning, communication, mood, and behaviour. It's the final one that scares me. Altered visual perception was also in there, but I don't know what that means and have no appetite to find out.

I also have no appetite to find out if I ever get to the point of being unable to remember my family, including my grandchildren. In my fifth year with dementia, I can still meet the requirements of reading, writing and, God knows, speaking. Dorothea will attest to my talking abilities.

Brain health is also maintained through diet and social activities. I'm giving myself an A-plus on all that. And I am enjoying life. But it will end; I am eighty-six, after all. So, I am left with thinking about my wife and how she manages it all. She will manage.

We had a wonderful visit with Geraldine Gunn from Newfoundland. Her late husband was a wonderful friend for years. Gerry, after mourning her loss, got on with her life, becoming a wonderful model for those with a tragic loss. For Dorothea, it was a wonderful break [in] her routine of keeping an eye on me. I was delighted to see them go "twacking"—which means looking around the stores.

I am convinced Dorothea can handle that.

Experts write that the brain is like a muscle that needs exercise. I think I'm up for that.

I will have no trouble remembering that visit from Gerry. It was inevitable, I suppose, that I would think of my own longevity.

I am convinced Dorothea, a strong woman, will be able to get on with her life when mine ends. Better if one of us has to get dementia that it be me. I don't think I would have the strength of will to continue without her. Years ago, I would tell her she had to let me die first because I couldn't live without her.

Dorothea has had to live with my dementia for five years and it makes me feel awful.

I think I may be reading too much about dementia. I see articles everywhere. Having said that, I am writing about it myself. The reactions I get suggest the public appreciates my efforts.

A headline in this paper read: "Don't Dehumanize People with Dementia." I must say, I have never felt dehumanized. The story was written by the Alzheimer Society's communications coordinator.

Those with dementia are told to ensure their rights are protected. The article says people with dementia deserve a good quality of life and to face less stigma. I am satisfied that I haven't faced that kind of a situation. I am pleased [the *Chronicle Herald*] gives me space to write. For me, it keeps the fog away.

Meanwhile [I] have decided to devote my next column to Dorothea. I hope she is okay with that.

57

My Anchor throughout My Life

Published March 25, 2019

This column is offered with a reluctant okay from the woman it is about.

Readers will notice that Dorothea plays a major role in all of my columns. I have decided to devote this column to tell you more about her.

A long time ago, my friend John Lewis told me about a young woman he met at university. Dorothea lived in Portugal Cove, NL, at the time. It's a small village outside St. John's. Her father drove her to Memorial University and she took the bus home.

I sought her out. I know she didn't seek me out. It was my early days at the CBC. Who would have thought that this young woman would become my anchor throughout my life? This column is intended to let you learn more about this wonderful woman, wonderful wife, wonderful mother, and wonderful nana.

I first started courting her when she was seventeen and I was an awkward twenty-two. Three years later, in 1958, we married. We cut short our honeymoon (we got bored) to move into our comfy little apartment. And on we went.

I have no idea if I was a good husband, but I knew I had a wonderful wife. Who would have thought that she would be burdened with a demented me in her eighties? How fortunate was I to have her with me.

Since we married, we have lived in four provinces while I was with the CBC: Newfoundland, Nova Scotia, Alberta, and Ontario (Toronto), as well as Manhattan, of all places. She never complained about the moves, even when we moved to New York so I could take a one-year job offer at the United Nations General Assembly newsroom.

UN staff said they had an apartment for us. They didn't. As it happened, Sheila, our first child, was an infant in a basket. We were left with hailing a taxi. As luck should have it, the driver said he knew of a place on Long Island that housed UN employees. Not a single complaint from Dorothea. One would think she would want to head home.

We had a bit of good luck. Others renting in the building included a couple from Newfoundland. And they had a child. They would look after Sheila while Dorothea toured Manhattan.

After I returned to CBC St. John's, I got another attack of wander-lust. I thought of exchanging jobs with a guy at CBC Edmonton just for the excitement of it. To cut the deal, we approached the CBC about funding our flights. They agreed and off we went with our three children in tow. We exchanged houses and Dorothea went for it.

I also worked in Toronto and, of course, Halifax. That's the kind of woman you read about in my columns. How lucky I was to have her agree to marry me and how grateful I am that John Lewis tipped me off about this wonderful teenager.

We now have six grandchildren, four of them in the neighbour-hood. So I don't get as much attention.

I think you've got a good idea of the kind of woman Dorothea was and still is.

58

For the Snowbound, Spring Offers a New Lease on Life

Published April 22, 2019

"Spring has sprung, the grass has riz. I wonder where the birdies is?" Or to borrow Martin Luther King's words: "Free at last, free at last." Seems a bit of an extreme welcome to spring but it gives me a new lease on life. Even to sit on the front deck and wave to neighbours is relaxing.

They may wonder why I'm waving. I had a little taste of it recently. Carol came to take me out for a sidewalk walk with my trusty walker. It was the first time since winter started. Of course, I do get out during the winter, but it is often a struggle for Dorothea to get me down the back steps, over icy patches to the car. Readers may think I'm exaggerating. Evoking King may seem a little extreme, I guess. The winter weather allowed me only rare trips to the gym. Dayna must have been bereft.

Back to dementia. Every day I come across more and more stories about dementia. Some are hard to believe. I should hold back on reading such stories, but the journalist in me pushes on.

In one story I read that opening your curtains could help. As it happens, we have a large living room window looking out over our front deck. Lo and behold, Dorothea just happens to do that to bring more natural light in. It does help, because it gets me out of my comfy den where I spend most of my time when I am not in bed.

I've also read that there is a way to put the unaffected parts of my brain to take up the slack and work harder. There is even talk of wearable cameras to record brain transplants. Sounds far-fetched.

I guess I should lay back and relax from reading that kind of stuff. But there is lots of humour in my house. There are times when, I'm told, I ask the same questions twice within minutes.

A friend of Dorothea called her recently from Florida. After reading one of my columns, she noted I had said Dorothea had been caring for me for five years. The friend called to say it's been a lot longer than five years.

Joshing me about my dementia, even from family, is not out of order. Even the grandchildren kid me about my memory lapses. We can't be serious all the time. A little jab here and there seems appropriate for this grandad.

So we will soon be able to spend time at Peter and Carol's cottage in Northport and visit with our friends the Letchers. That might seem like a small thing, but it's essential for a guy who's been snowbound for months.

59

"Fun bedlam" Had by All at Irish Music Gathering

Published May 27, 2019

I was somewhat premature when I announced in my last column that spring had sprung. The next day, the car was buried in snow. I don't want to blame anyone for this, but it is tempting to blame it on Ryan. He used to do the forecasting in my native Newfoundland, one of the hardest spots on Earth to predict the weather. So I expect better weather from him.

However, he was joined by Cindy Day in [the *Chronicle Herald*]. So, I guess I'll blame both of them if the forecast doesn't hold.

I have read a lot lately about dealing with dementia. My next column, if [the *Chronicle Herald*] obliges, will deal with my escape from my homebound winter and my reaction to warm weather. I am a home prisoner in winter.

In the interim, we had a wonderful visit from our Irish friends by way of Toronto, Bob and Christine Culbert.

Bob worked with me at the CBC. As expected, Bob brought along some "sucky" Irish music. So, we gathered the MacKays and other friends for a singalong. It was bedlam, but fun bedlam. As it happens, I knew a lot of the songs, so I was able to insert my dulcet tones into the songs. Even the MacKays pretended to be Irish.

I danced with daughter-in-law, Carol, and we made a handsome couple. It was one of those old-fashioned dances where you actually have contact with your partner. Peter was out of town, so we were safe. Dorothea enjoyed the show.

I promised not to use the "Mercy Convent dip" while dancing. I won't describe that fancy move, lest we shock tender souls. Christine took a photo and sent it out to all and sundry.

As I've noted in earlier columns, we have had wonderful visits from friends since my diagnosis. Bob and Christine are the only ones who brought music. I hope the neighbours appreciated it.

I have mentioned in other columns how important it is for the two of us to have visitors. My next column will talk about the wonderful family gathering we had over Easter.

It was announced in [the *Chronicle Herald*] recently that researcher Ian Pottie has found a $710,000 superconducting magnet to explore the brain. Ouch! He calls it a game changer. He will be assisted by Sultan Darvesh of Dalhousie University, whom Dorothea and I have already met and talked to. As I remember, he had on display a bunch of brains to point out the troubled ones.

He did ask if he could have mine when I'm finished, and I have told him to go for it.

60

Dorothea Is, after All, My Memory

Published June 17, 2019

"Kindness" is an oft-used word but carries a mountain of meanings for Dorothea and me. I witnessed it just recently on two occasions.

As Dorothea was helping me off the back deck, a man we had never met, who was working on a neighbour's property, hurried over and offered me a strong shoulder to use getting me down to the car and went back to work. We never caught his name. But he had parting words: "If there were no old people, young people would learn nothing." Then off he went. So there!

On the same day, while out to the gym, it happened again. I began to feel faint and thought I may fall. Dale and Dayna from the gym saw what was happening, hurried over with water, and helped Dorothea get me to the car.

They waited until I was nestled in and all comfy. I was back at the gym the next day and a cautious Dayna adjusted the regimen just in case I repeated my show. People we don't know will stop us on the street to ask how we are doing. Strangers being kind. And of course, Peter, Carol, and Donna play a major role in keeping us engaged. Joann, the wonderful woman who comes bi-weekly to help me clean house, is also a wonderful inspiration.

In my columns, I try to transmit into print what is going on in my mind. In idle moments, and there are many, I fake it that I am doing some deep thinking. Doesn't fool Dorothea. She is, after all, my memory.

Meanwhile, there is lots of research going on to figure out what causes dementia.

Professor Ian Pottie of Mount Saint Vincent University is researching dementia and is excited about using a nuclear magnetic resonance spectrometer for his research. He calls it a game changer. As someone with dementia, I am cautious about a "game changer," whatever that is. It all sounds too complicated for me to understand, but I am willing to volunteer to help. I think.

Respected columnist Andre Picard writes that we can delay the onset of dementia: avoid inactivity (hmmm), obesity (hardly), write (I do), play music (I don't), be socially engaged (I am).

Our neighbours across the lane, the Johnsons, are also kind to us. They keep an eye on us. We know they will help if needed.

That's enough of all that. We will soon have all but one of our entire family together again for Mother's Day when Sheila comes to visit with son Patrick. Gabrielle couldn't make it this time.

When Sheila comes in, all the lights go on. And we will all be together again. Peter, Carol, Amber, and David; Donna, Seamus and Molly, and Sheila's Patrick. A well-deserved celebration of Dorothea's wonderful contribution to all our lives—Mother's Day.

61

A Family Frolic at the Cottage

Published July 15, 2019

What a party we had at Jack Lake at the Culberts' cottage north of Toronto.

Bob and Christine Culbert invited all of our available family. We wondered how we could all be accommodated at a cottage. Some cottage—bedrooms and bathrooms had been added in an adjoining cottage. I'm lost for words—not really—to describe the time we had at the cottage. But don't panic. It's a temporary loss of words, of course.

The cottage party included two granddads, (Bob and me); two nanas, Dorothea and Christine; three mothers, Alison and Donna and Sheila; a dad, Jeff; a son, Andrew; and a scattering of grandsons and granddaughters, Seamus and Molly MacInnes, Maeve and Dylan, Patrick and Gabrielle.

Andrew's friend, another Allison (with two Ls), was there too and winked at me throughout the evening. Dorothea was not offended. Andrew was bemused.

You would not describe Bob or me as handymen. There was a problem with no warm water. Jeff wandered in and flicked a switch. The hot water appeared. Alison and Jeff are both physicians but have proved to be handy people.

My grandchildren saw the need for keeping an eye on me, lest I fall and put a damper on the event. Gabrielle and Seamus are always on the alert when I am around.

Bob, as expected, brought music along and everyone got on the floor, except yours truly. Dorothea feared I'd fall. Andrew's Allison looked seriously disappointed that she couldn't have a dance with me.

The grandchildren had a grand time frolicking in the lake. It's just as well I am beyond frolicking. Or maybe not, in my condition. Christine had long expressed a wish that both families could get together. She got it done, although Peter and Carol were in Europe.

I get to use a wheelchair in airports. The flight attendants got me in and out of the airplanes. I made that fun, and the attendants enjoyed it. On departing the plane in Halifax, I travelled through a crowd of passengers waiting to get on the flight. I pretended I believed they were a welcome-home committee and thanked them profusely. They got it. I never fail to embarrass Dorothea, who was pushing me.

One would think she should be used to my shenanigans.

My good friend Jo Ann MacKay has suggested that I spend my next column explaining how I am doing instead of what I am doing. She believes it would be helpful to those who have been diagnosed.

62

How Dementia Handles Me

Published August 12, 2019

A close friend suggested to me that, because I write so much about how I handle dementia, I should devote a column on how dementia handles me. I don't know where to start. Dorothea and my family will have to help me there.

The most obvious issue is balance, and that attracts the attention of family. I use a walker when I am out and about, and a clumping cane when I am walking around the house. She knows when I am coming. Taking the stairs, I need rails for both hands. I have to watch my language when I go on about that.

When Dorothea goes out without me, I ask where she is going and when she will return. I worry about the traffic. If I hear a siren, I immediately assume the worst. In a case like that, she may text me with a reassurance. There's an old song about "looking on the sunny side of life." I gotta get back to that.

I think my temperament is fine. I don't pity myself, but I regret how it has affected Dorothea. My mood doesn't alter when my memory lets me down. In fact, I am quite neighbourly and often, while at a restaurant, I strike up a conversation with other diners. They usually have a few questions for Dorothea. Because of the way I react to my condition, strangers feel they can approach us with some questions.

At lunch recently we sat across from two elderly men. I learned they were two old friends who enjoyed chatting. I was curious about how long they were friends so, as expected, I started a conversation with them. One of them recognized me and asked some questions. As usual I replied with alacrity. They also had questions for Dorothea.

I now have a medical alert system if I fall. I wear a gizmo around my neck and a receiver of sorts inside. This is one thing I hope never happens.

63

Yes, Really—I Do Write This Column

Published September 3, 2019

Before I begin my usual column, I would like to address the concerns of a *Chronicle Herald* subscriber who feels I don't actually write these columns.

I do, of course. I think perhaps I'm still able to due to a number of things, including a very early diagnosis and also, likely, taking a drug during a research project for three years.

Dorothea noted a difference in me when the drug was suddenly stopped, although it seemed I was still able to write. On one of our first visits to the memory clinic I learned that often many people with dementia retain a reservoir of ability in areas at which they once excelled.

Although I am very grateful I can still write, I am deteriorating in other ways.

My memory loss, for example, is most noticeable. I can no longer follow my BBC mysteries. I am unsure how to get places. I sometimes can't remember conversations I have had a day or two ago. I am now physically frail, but that way I don't have to do anything around the house. Despite all that, I am so grateful to be able to engage in everyday activities, albeit it with help from family and friends.

The "veil of tears" is not going to overcome me. My thanks go to Dorothea, my family, and many friends. Peter, Donna, and Carol never locked me out, as they say. Sheila lives in Toronto and stays in touch.

Granddaughter Molly wanted to have her birthday party with Nana and Grandad and her friends. Molly's friends knew of my dementia and were quite comfortable. It certainly made me feel younger. Without family and friends my lot would not be a happy one.

Dorothea went home to St. John's to see her old friend whose husband had died. It gave her a welcome break from keeping an eye on me, albeit with help from family and friends again. I had a wonderful experience recently with a young woman at Peter and Carol's home. Maddy Hiscock is Carol's niece. Her mother is Carol's twin, Cheryl Hiscock.

One might expect a young woman to be a little hesitant chatting up an octogenarian with dementia. Not at all. Maddy chose to sit by me at dinner and we talked about everything but my mental health problem. I fell in love with Maddy. Peter was there to entertain us, so I didn't get all the attention.

Maddie's friend Liam was also with us and appeared to enjoy Peter's humour. Carol rolls her eyes when Peter is performing.

I had another wonderful experience with Donna's long-time friend Liz. She has experienced dementia in her family. At times I pretended to forget her name. Anything for a laugh. My mother used to call me a lackadaisical omadhaun.

While at Peter and Carol's cottage in Northport we dropped in on good friends Linda and Owen Letcher, where cookies and coffee awaited. They are the parents of Dale, who operates the gym that keeps me so fit. Okay, not that fit. Owen enjoys a CBC pension as well. He did the useful stuff as a technician while I lolled about as a talker.

While Dorothea was away, Donna came over and slept to keep an eye on me. She put a limit on my Manhattans. I was surprised how much I missed Dorothea while she was gone. When I was working with the CBC I travelled a lot, leaving my wife to look after the family.

Donna was wonderful. She spent the nights in our house and took some time off work to be there with me. She snuck me a Manhattan when the coast was clear.

Donna knew how much I enjoyed Mahone Bay, so we (she) drove down and shopped at Wile's Bakery and chatted with the owner, Elspeth. It was noted that she and Donna were widows, making do.

64

My Granddaughter Molly Brings Her Birthday to Me

Published October 15, 2019

As expected, family came to the rescue when the hurricane was predicted. Peter and Carol secured our outdoor furniture and they and Donna kept an eye on us. Grandson Seamus took down our hanging baskets.

My granddaughter's birthday got a cursory glance in an earlier column. It deserves more.

Dorothea and I were paid a huge tribute recently when Molly MacInnes told us she wanted to celebrate her nineteenth birthday in our house. Molly and I have had a special bond for many of those years. She and her brother, Seamus, lost their dad some years ago and their mom, Donna, took the reins. Molly and her granddad seem to have a special bond. Hugs are always offered when we are together.

So, in they came, Molly and six of her girlfriends. No boys. The seven young women were quite relaxed.

Donna decorated the living room with balloons and frillies. Molly's friends, a "gaggle of gigglers," knew of my dementia, and I made a few jokes about it to be sure they relaxed. My appearance at the party didn't seem to be a damper on the doings. There was no talk about boys.

We had a nice lunch in the dining room where the laughter never ceased. You could see they were still close friends from school. Seamus and I were the only men at the party. We did nothing more than laugh.

Molly is of an age when she goes "downtown" in the evenings. I think one of the teens admitted she was too young for a pub crawl. So off they went, giggling all the way.

As I noted in earlier columns, Dorothea and I are lucky octogenarians. We older folk have our laughs. Recently, in the car, I noted that my hearing aids are working well.

"What?" she replied. A howl of laughter followed. Later, as she was plugging in my hearing aids, I told her there was a mysterious noise in one of them. It was the kettle boiling. Even just with the two of us together we still share a lot of laughter.

I'm not making any of this up. Some experts write that dementia brings depression. Not in this house. For a guy with dementia, I am able to enjoy myself a lot. All thanks to a wonderful wife and a wonderful family.

Recently, I was visited by a Fardy I didn't know. More on that in a future column, if [the *Chronicle Herald*] obliges.

Looking up at my bookshelf in the den recently I noticed a book I didn't even know I had. *When Someone You Know Has Dementia*. Really! Author June Andrews offered *Practical Advice for Family Caregivers*. Dame Judi Dench wrote the foreword. With all due respect, Dorothea and my family know well how to handle that disease.

So far, my journey has not been difficult, though it has turned Dorothea's life around.

65

My Newsy Mom Loved Hearing Me on the CBC

Published November 12, 2019

I t was suggested to me that I should write about my mother, Mary "Mame" (Doody) Fardy, backbone of our large family of four boys and two girls. She was born in Carbonear, Conception Bay, Newfoundland and Labrador.

The best story I have is about our youngest, Mary, who had Down syndrome. Instead of keeping her home, Mom sent her off to the girls' school. Her intention was to introduce Mary to the real world and not hide her away. Years later when I was walking with her, a flock of young students would say hi to Mary. They were in her class in school. Of course, Mary didn't advance and soon came home to stay. But in a small neighbourhood everyone knew her.

Mary changed my name to Darce because she had difficulty with Gerard.

My brother Paul, who went on to university, said he never passed in a report without showing it first to Mom. My father, Hugh, a quiet man, had little to do with raising his family. A telegrapher, he walked to work early every morning, walked home for dinner, then back down, and home for supper. His proudest boast was my brother Hugh, a local star athlete. My brother Frank, the only modest one among the four of us, married a nurse and they had a flock of seven kids who produced fourteen grandchildren. I sometimes see the name Frank Fardy on Facebook and wonder who owns him.

I'm the only survivor in the family, at eighty-seven.

Mom was a newsy woman who worked at the *Daily News* and was delighted when I got a job at the CBC during the pre-television days. I would sometimes offer a report for the eleven o'clock (P.M.) news with no guarantee it would be used. It was "on spec," as they say. But Mom would stay up with me to hear me if it were used. She was puffed up when my strong Newfoundland accent was heard. I don't think Dad stayed up to hear me. Mom would be up at six to prepare breakfast for her flock.

I always wore hand-me-downs from my brothers, often with patches in the seats of the pants. When standing in school I would keep my back to the wall. Mom's response: "They are clean, aren't they?"

The four boys would traipse down to Aunt Annie's for a bath every Saturday. I don't know how we managed that. She and Uncle Bob had no children. I remember Uncle Bob reminding me to chew my milk, whatever that meant.

And I remember a Christmas when we couldn't afford a turkey. Dad went off to a downtown raffle and returned home triumphantly holding a turkey over his head. He had won it.

Anyway, I think Mom helped me grow up and attain some success.

Sheila, Peter, and Donna didn't get enough time to know Nana Fardy. Nana Neary, Dorothea's mother, was around a lot longer for my family to get to know her. She was, of course, a lot younger than Mom and I don't think the two Moms knew each other.

A Newfoundland comedian, Tommy Sexton, said, "I'm going to heaven 'cause Mom said I was." So, there you are. The power of Moms.

The other wonderful Mom I admire is, of course, Dorothea.

66

Winter's Arrival Limits My Mobility

Published December 16, 2019

B ack when the Catholic mass was in Latin, one of the prominent prayers was "*De Profundis Clamavi Ad Te Domine*," which translates as, "Out of the Depths I Have Cried to Thee, Oh Lord." Even though I have been dealing with dementia for seven or so years, there has never been any despair. In fact, there has been a lot of laughter at my own memory lapses.

Recently, when it was flu shot time, Dorothea laid on an appointment for me at my doctor's office for the next morning. I was ready and able. When we got in the car the next morning, I forgot about the doctor and asked where we were going. When she told me, I broke into laughter, and was still laughing when we entered the doctor's office.

When Christmas came into view I asked if I could do anything to help. I interpreted a grim look in reply as a suggestion I stay out of the way.

Dorothea's brother visited recently from Newfoundland, God's country. Family and friends were alerted because Doug always brings fresh cod and cooks for family and friends.

Thirteen of us crowded around the table to partake, including, of course, Wayne and Jo Ann MacKay. Two other friends we had not seen in a long time, Art and Bethany, joined us.

Here's a good one. The telephone (remember them?) rang and I answered it. It was for Dorothea but I didn't know how to put it on hold. On the other hand, I mastered texting, so there!

On a more serious note, perhaps, Dorothea and I took in most of the Trump impeachment hearing. Most of that was laughable, though without that intention.

Life becomes more difficult for me and the family when winter arrives. Dorothea helps me over the steps to the car. I won't attempt that when there is snow on the ground. If I have to go out, Peter or Carol or Seamus or Molly or David will carry me out! Entertainment for the neighbours. Winter brings many "stay at home" days for me. Given my lack of walking skills, nurse Carol has given me a chart of exercises to follow to keep me moving, at least in the house.

The Alzheimer Society reports that many people with dementia try to hide it. That is sad, especially since the Society has so many things to offer in coping with dementia. A recent story in [the *Chronicle Herald*] urges readers not to "dehumanize people with dementia." I have never experienced that. In fact, when Dorothea and I are out in a restaurant, frequently other diners will come by to wish us the best.

I hope others living with dementia will talk to others about it. There is no shame in it.

2020

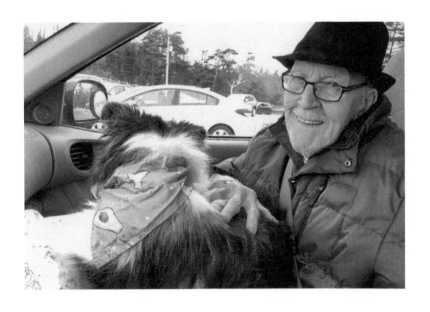

67

All Aboard for a Big Family Christmas

Published January 27, 2020

Gabrielle, Patrick, Seamus, Molly, Amber, and David, our grandchildren, were with Nana and Granddad and their parents for Christmas Day. The dining room table was extended to accommodate them and their parents, Sheila, Peter and Carol, Donna and, of course, their proud grandparents. What more could Dorothea and I ask for?

Dorothea, of course, gets ready in November, knitting Christmas stockings for the new arrivals of friends and baking fruitcakes for family and friends. They numbered eight this year, some delivered by mail to friends.

As for the new arrivals, the babies' names are sewn into the stockings. One of the names was Alexander. That took a while. The stockings are big enough so the babies can fit inside them.

She also decorates the tree and the living room. Some of the tree decorations are over sixty years old. You may ask what I do to help prepare. Precious little, as they say. I'd be called a slouch in Newfoundland, just sitting in my comfy den chair. And I am a lot older than the decorations.

Sheila lives in Toronto and came down with her two kids, Gabrielle and Patrick. It's a command performance for me. It wouldn't be Christmas without the flock here and we all admit Sheila brings a certain glow, a joie de vivre, the entire Christmas week. The sun sets a little earlier when she leaves and takes her two with her.

It's a rare occasion when all six grandchildren gather in our den while the rest of us sit in the living room discussing world affairs. From the laughter we hear there is no doubt they love and enjoy each other. But you can't have Christmas without winter. The snow falls and, as the song says, I don't get around much anymore in the winter. It's too much to ask of Dorothea to help me to the car when the trip could be a slippery one. The neighbours must be entertained watching family help the old guy to the car.

You may find this a weird wish, but I'd like to be out shovelling snow.

We entered a new year as I was writing all this. I will turn eighty-eight in a few months, outliving my three brothers by many years.

I have what might be called a staggering gait, even while walking around the house. The trusty cane is essential. I have promised not to act flahoolick, [*sic*: flockahoolic] a word my mother used a lot in Newfoundland when someone was being foolish.

So there!

68
Fending off the Idle Mind

Unpublished. February 2020

"So how are you doing?" I am often asked. I have to think about that. There is no change in my dementia so that question should be put to Dorothea.

I know there is no cure so I know I will never be out driving the car or dropping into a restaurant or shop on my own. Or even walking around the block on my own. I'd like to try that along with my walker but that can't happen for obvious reasons. So, I spend my winters reading in the den, and watching the news. A break for me will come in the summer when I can sit on the porch in my deck chair. My mother used to say, "An idle mind is the devil's workshop." So I had better keep reading and offering up my columns.

It is worth noting that at eighty-seven (eighty-eight in May) none of my three brothers and two sisters lived to be that age. I read the other day a story about what is called "Generation X" or "boomer" or "millennial." I don't know what class I belong in.

Talk about nice gestures! There are two nearby restaurants we usually patronize. When the waiters see us struggle in, an employee will help us steer my walker to our table. Not shy, I usually raise my hands in victory when I finally perch. Dorothea usually raises her eyebrows. The Esquire on the Bedford highway is our frequent target for lunch because it seems to be frequented by older folks and is near the home we raised our family in.

My target now is to avoid pessimism. It doesn't threaten until I go to bed and there are no distractions. There is no cure for dementia, but pessimism doesn't help. I often have grandkids in the house to cheer me up. They are all aware of my problem and help me soldier on.

Here's one for the books. I picked up a *Maclean's* magazine the other day and was well into it when I noticed it was dated July 2019. Go figure! Newsy guy?...Sure.

As I was completing this column I learned of the death back home of my sister-in-law, Mary (Howlett) Fardy, the widow of my brother Frank, who died some years ago. I used to phone her from time to time to chat. They led a quiet life even with seven children in eight years. She tended to all their needs, including checking their homework, while continuing her nursing career. Frank was known as the only modest one among my family.

My three brothers died many years ago.

69

Donna Drives Me Everywhere

Published March 2, 2020

My daughter Donna, the youngest of our three, knows I like driving around with her. Although she works, she manages to fit me into her busy schedule to take me to places around Halifax that I haven't been since I was diagnosed with dementia and stopped driving. She's the mother of Seamus and Molly, whose dad died some years ago.

Donna is a good friend as well as a wonderful daughter. For winter driving she turns on the heat under my butt so it's nice and comfy. We also try to find a nice restaurant in the area we are visiting. Being me, I chat with people in the restaurant. One customer, a woman of a certain age, came in and I spoke to her. I told her about my dementia. She came to that familiar restaurant, I think, because it was a friendly place for her. I think she may live alone.

Donna also comes by to put our garbage out.

Daughter-in-law, Carol, lives across the street and has been available to provide two octogenarians with valuable health care advice. When Dorothea had occasion to visit her doctor, Carol went along to help her understand exactly what was going on. Both of us found that very comforting. Carol has also shown me how to exercise my arms, hips, and legs while sitting down. When summer arrives and I can get out with my walker, I know that Donna or Carol will walk with me around the block, and I can wave to my fans.

If you know Lewis Carroll's poem "The Walrus and the Carpenter," you know the passage: "'The time has come,' the Walrus said, 'To talk of many things: Of shoes—and ships—and sealing-wax—Of cabbages—and kings—...'"

That would be me. Another saying: "An idle mind is the devil's workshop." My mother used to tell me that. My mind is damaged a bit but not idle. Dorothea wishes my tongue was idle more.

I read two or three magazines including *Maclean's* and *Zoomer* and, of course, *The Walrus*. I also read *Downhome*, and you can guess where that is published. A companion magazine specializes in news from Labrador.

I read somewhere recently a story promoting "Fifteen things you can do to prevent dementia." Too late for me. Dealing with dementia is something Dorothea and I are masters at.

To quote another poem: "When things go wrong as they sometimes will, when the road you are walking is all uphill...Rest if you want, but don't you quit." So there.

I hesitate to promote a restaurant, but we found one on the Bedford Highway (the Esquire) that provides easy access to a guy with a walker.

A sad note: Recently, my sister-in-law Mary Howlett Fardy died in St. John's. Mary and my late brother Frank raised seven children.

70

Don't Get Around Much Anymore

Unpublished. May 8, 2020

Years ago there was a popular song that used the phrase "don't get around much anymore." I haven't been getting around since my diagnosis with dementia but now with the arrival of COVID-19 I am joined by millions of people. At this time no one will be getting around until the virus runs its course. Everyone in the world has to deal with it. It means for us no visitors to our home and none by us to Peter and Carol or Donna, all of whom live nearby.

We are told that seniors are most at risk. Dorothea and I do not regard as ourselves as seniors, just parents and grandparents. And it is family drop-ins we miss most. We miss the family visit.

We have good friends who volunteer to shop for us, leaving the groceries and other necessities within our reach on the back deck. Daughter-in-law, Carol, also lets Dorothea know when she is going out for groceries. And of course, daughter Donna is always in touch. I call Donna every morning when I get out of bed.

Fortunately, Dorothea and I are devoted news hawks.

Dorothea is also an avid reader. I nod off unless the book is a real dandy. I'm told I have a vague memory of events today but remember well the first twenty years of my life. Go figure! After that, not so much.

I've already disclosed that my wife does everything that needs to be done while I am watching television, CBC of course, but also PBS.

Dorothea is also bemused when I sit in the den and watch a program I've already seen.

Luckily, we still find things to laugh about. And we both anxiously await the time family and friends can drop in, but there's also room for laughter. I had my wristwatch on backwards recently and it appeared to have gained half an hour in a few seconds. I can be watching a television program and am told I watched it earlier. On the other side, when I start to watch a new program, I am convinced I saw it before—however, I have no idea what the ending is!

Recently, Donna visited with her two, Seamus and Molly, and called us from the front walk for us to come out and sit on the front deck while they stayed on the walk. It is a simple gesture, but it means a lot to us. Also, recently we got a surprise at our back door. We heard people outside and found Peter and Carol with their daughter, Amber, and son, David. We chatted and waved from the back deck.

As a former journalist I was apolitical, but I can't resist praising our Prime Minister for being so open and accountable. Our own Premier has also made a huge contribution to encourage us.

Good weather is taking its time, but I should get out on my deck to read and relax...while sipping a Manhattan. That should get a visit from Wayne!

71

A Day Trip to the Cottage; No Tools Required

Unpublished. July 9, 2020

On a sunny day recently, Dorothea and I thought it was a good day for a quick visit to Peter and Carol at their cottage in Northport. A kind of drop-in to sit on the deck and enjoy the view of the water. The cottage is on a slope that reveals other cottages on the shoreline. It turned out to be a party for which ten people turned up. All of them were nearby cottagers and many of them, Carol's relatives. Her family had a cottage there and that attracted their children to do the same. Among the bunch were Carol's identical twin, Cheryl, and her husband, Rob. They live in New Brunswick. The COVID barrier had just been lifted.

I was all puffed up by the attention until I noticed they came to watch Peter and Carol build a shed. For some reason Peter did not need my help. His niece Molly is a new graduate in carpentry, getting honours at NSCC. I couldn't help her with her homework!

As we were leaving the cottage, Carol's sister Liz, who is a physiotherapist, showed me some exercises which could help strengthen the muscles in my arms and legs. I will try to do as she said. I once went to the gym regularly but became discouraged when I fell on my face and had to be helped to the car.

I had my eighty-eighth birthday on May 15, but no party. At eighty-eight, I am a hop, skip, and jump from ninety. Time to start thinking of old age. Even though I have been dealing with dementia for nearly a decade, I must say I have a wonderful life. My own family makes a huge contribution. Sheila, Peter and Carol, and Donna are always there for encouragement.

Four of our six grandchildren live in our neighbourhood. The other two are in Toronto. We can FaceTime Sheila and her two so we can see each other and even get a virtual tour of Sheila's newly renovated house. Donna, Seamus, and Molly visited at a distance and Molly brought me a birthday cake, which we ate on the deck, being careful to keep the right distance. Peter, Carol, Amber, and David were at their cottage, but came a few days later and visited from the steps to the back deck.

I think readers will agree that while there is no cure for dementia, there is little reason I should be depressed.

- 30 -

Epilogue

T hat was that last column my father was able to complete (with a lot of help from my mother). Somewhat poignantly, it was about an experience from which he derived great joy. It's not that he went "cold turkey" and decided to stop writing. For much of the seventeen-month period between that final column and his death, he retained an interest in writing. By this time, however, it was obvious to those of us around him that he was not able to see a column through from idea to completion. We did not discourage him from writing, but neither did we encourage it. Whatever he wanted to talk about or spend time on—whatever made him happy—was good enough for us.

During the last two years of his life, Dad's condition continued to deteriorate. His need for physical supports and almost constant supervision took its toll on both him and those closest to him, and his quality of life was in steady decline. His mood, while still often upbeat, became more volatile and difficult to predict. He became emotional and maudlin more frequently. We were told that all of this is common among those living with dementia.

Over his final year, he became more and more concerned about "being a burden," especially to our mother, and almost no amount of assurance otherwise could divert him from that preoccupation.

Despite these inevitabilities, he remained engaged and engaging, right to the end. He never wanted to reach the point where he did not know his family, and his exit from this world had him fully aware that he was surrounded by those who loved him. He passed with tremendous grace.

We have learned through this experience that every story is different. This is just one person's and one family's story. Every case of dementia and Alzheimer's manifests and presents in its own unique way. There is nothing the reader can take from these pages that will predict anyone else's path.

However, by understanding that every situation is unique, caregivers can focus on supporting their family member in the way that makes sense to them, without the pressure of feeling like there is only one right way to provide such support.

For what it is worth, what worked best for us was trying to retain as much normalcy as possible (easy at the beginning, but less so later on), without denying the fact of the disease. As is clearly apparent from his writing, frequent socialization and humour were key ingredients.

Peter Fardy, July 2024

Fardy, Gerard J. "Darce"

May 15, 1932–March 12, 2022

Darce Fardy, *eighty-nine, died the way he lived—with dignity—on Saturday, March 12, 2022, at home in Halifax. He left this life surrounded by his loving family, at the time and place of his own choosing, and fully at peace. But only after a toast, a Manhattan, a laugh, a cry, and a rousing chorus of Ode to Newfoundland. We should all have such great fortune.*

He was born May 15, 1932, in St. John's, NL. His given name was Gerard, but no one ever called him that. Even he was not absolutely sure where "Darce" came from. When pressed, he would recite his full name as "Gerard James Robert Irish-Nick Cooper-Conn Aloysius Gonzaga Rumbia Fardy."

"Darce" it was, then.

After attending and (by some accounts) graduating from St. Bonaventure's College (St. Bon's) he ascended from the role of senior altar boy at the Basilica and, lacking more compelling prospects, packed it off to upstate New York to join the Order of the Irish Christian Brothers. Demonstrating limited creative range, he took the name "Bonaventure." His proclivity for irreverence, humour, and mischief was sufficiently disruptive to see him soon spirited away in the middle of the night and put on the train back home. That signalled the end of both Brother Bonaventure and his vows of poverty, chastity, and obedience, for which his future spouse and offspring remain eternally grateful (especially with respect to the first two).

Undeterred by this unceremonious defrocking, he fell into a job at the fledgling Canadian Broadcasting Corporation in St. John's, only three years after anything in Newfoundland was labelled "Canadian." There, he worked his way through

the newsroom and soon became the first national news reporter for CBC television in the tenth province. His was the voice of
Newfoundland to the rest of Canada, reporting on any and all
matters of provincial or national import. Prime Minister John
Diefenbaker once pronounced "all I hear of Newfoundland
comes from my good friend Darce Fardy."

In 1954 Darce was introduced to seventeen-year-old
Dorothea Jean Neary of Portugal Cove by a mutual friend. His
dogged, if sometimes awkward, pursuit eventually bore fruit
when she agreed to marry him in 1958. Reflective of his pledge
to keep Dorothea "in the lifestyle to which she had become
accustomed," the published wedding announcement reported
that "Mr. and Mrs. Fardy will be spending their honeymoon on
a "driving holiday." And off they went to Makinsons (pop. circa
450), an hour's drive west.

Darce's career with the CBC led him into increasingly
interesting and challenging roles, including a stint at the
United Nations in New York, in the newsroom in Edmonton,
as Director of Television in St. John's and Halifax, and eventually to network HQ in Toronto, where he served as Head of
Current Affairs, overseeing programs such as The Journal,
The Fifth Estate, and Marketplace (to name a few), as well as
all documentary productions, including many international
award–winners. He loved every job he had at the CBC and
retired in 1991.

For a period during his CBC career, Darce also served
part-time in the reserves as a Naval Lieutenant. Maritime
Command must have never felt so vulnerable. In 1979–80 he
was chosen to attend the National Defence College, based in
Kingston, ON, for a year of geo-political globe-trotting with
fifty other Canadian military officers and civilian leaders
strapped into a RCAF Hercules transport aircraft. They visited
six continents, meeting with government leaders from dozens
of countries.

Darce saw retirement as a word, not a state of being. He therefore accepted an appointment as the first Review Officer overseeing the Nova Scotia Freedom of Information and Protection of Privacy Act, where he drew both admiration and ire from elected officials and senior public servants, depending on whether they were the requestors or requestees of government-held information. He served in that role for eleven years, "re-retiring" in 2007. Still not prepared to step fully back, he founded the Nova Scotia Right to Know Coalition, an advocacy not-for-profit, which he ran from his home office—between the chest freezer and the furnace in the basement—for several years.

In 2013 Darce was awarded the Queen's Diamond Jubilee Medal in recognition of his commitment and contribution to public access to information. As someone who lived off the public purse his whole life, it seemed a delicious irony that he was nominated for this honour by the Canadian Taxpayer's Federation. A compliment if there ever was one.

Darce was diagnosed with Alzheimer's disease in 2013. To his credit, he immediately (and voluntarily) turned in his car keys and decided, as a former journalist, to share his story of living with dementia through a semi-regular column in the Halifax Chronicle Herald. *Thankfully, the disease progressed slowly enough that he was able to write the column, with increasing doses of intervention from editor-in-chief Dorothea, for many years. Countless friends and strangers commented on how much they appreciated this effort to both de-stigmatize the disease and give others dealing with it some comfort.*

Darce was predeceased by his parents, Hugh James Fardy and Mary (Doody) Fardy, older brothers Hugh, Frank, and Paul, older sister Margaret O'Brien, and his younger sister and favourite, Mary. It was left to him to turn out the lights as the last Fardy sibling to leave the party. He also lost his son-in-law, Donnie MacInnes, in 2010.

He is survived by his loving and medal-deserving wife of sixty-three years, Dorothea, who claims the secret to their long marriage was a husband who was away a lot. He will be greatly missed by his daughters Sheila and Donna, son, Peter (Carol), who, as children, could hardly contain themselves at the breakfast table in anticipation of their dad saying goodbye, pretending to miss the kitchen doorway, and walking into the wall. He did not disappoint.

Darce is also survived by six grandchildren, of whom he was very proud, and from whom he took great joy: Gabrielle and Patrick Emilien, Amber and David Fardy, and Seamus and Molly MacInnes. As Grandad, he took tremendous interest in their many academic, athletic, professional, and extra-curricular pursuits.

The family suggests that donations in Darce's memory, for those inclined, may be made to the Alzheimer Society of Nova Scotia, or to support Alzheimer's research at Dalhousie University.

Afterword

I am glad to have had the opportunity to read Darce's book and to reflect on the straightforward way in which he approached living with dementia. His forthrightness inspired me to accept the offer by the publisher to also write this short afterword. In many of the columns I wrote which accompanied Darce's writing, I had spoken of optimism that, in 2014, Nova Scotia would do better to plan for an ageing population, of which more people living with dementia would be an inevitable part. The publisher asked whether I felt that any of this had worked out.

Although the demographic projection proved true—we have many more Nova Scotians living with dementia now than we did a decade ago—largely, my optimism was misplaced. We fell well short of where we needed to be. I might offer, regarding my outlook, that I am a geriatrician—that is, an internal medicine specialist who has done an additional two years of training in the health care of older adults. Like most others of this cohort, I am constitutively a wary optimist. Also, I had reason to maintain a positive outlook: a newly elected government had commissioned a dementia strategy and had asked me to lead it.

I brought together an outstanding multidisciplinary panel of experts, each a pragmatist with a proven history of successful reform and advice to government. We consulted with a range of people who worked in the sector and knew well the lived experience of dementia—including by having lived it as patients or, more often, as caregivers. But it was not to be: the much-watered-down document we developed occupies an infinitely small space on the internet (novascotia.ca/dhw/dementia). From the 2015 Nova Scotia Dementia Strategy we saw some much-needed and welcome funding for the Alzheimer Society of Nova Scotia's important roles in advocacy and front-line advice and support. Still, the impact of the Dementia Strategy is about exactly proportionate to its size online.

Otherwise, much of what we had advocated for—better design of public space, more age-friendly housing, more dementia-friendly health care practice, and fewer perverse incentives in the design, implementation, measurement of, and funding for dementia care—remains untouched. Crushingly, this all comes on top of what is, at best, seriously stalled progress on treatment, with the Alzheimer's research community often simply tinkering with what has not worked.

And yet, I cannot be the enemy of hope. We see small signs that hint at real progress on the research front. And in Nova Scotia, despite the pandemic tragedies that were disproportionately experienced by people affected by dementia, it is easy to sense some progress. Some of this sensing is idiosyncratic: in my case, it depends on my now having a better view. In 2014 I was mostly a voice on the outside. A few years later, I was invited to become, as Darce might have put it, "part of the problem." For me, that meant joining the senior leadership team at what is now Nova Scotia Health.

In my role with the Frailty and Elder Care Network I am seeing the first hints of success after a mountain of work to make care better. As a lifelong Anglican, I've often remarked, half in jest and wholly in earnest, "I get resistance to change; it's how we roll." Still, it is something else to see just how beguiled we are by a status quo that often neither serves people who live with dementia well, nor their families. I see opportunities for change in how the present government is making room to hear from people who understand the system well—both providers and consumers. Time will tell whether this makes a lasting difference. For now, all I can say is that it feels much different from where we were a decade ago.

The lesson we should take from Darce Fardy's is that if dementia befalls us, we should aim to live as fully as we can. That means engaging now in what might prevent it or lessen its course: getting a timely and accurate diagnosis, being offered treatment, having the effect of treatment monitored, and making sure that people are there not just for us but for our families.

Mostly though, it means pushing hard to make things better.

Kenneth Rockwood, MD, February 2024

Further Information from the Alzheimer Society of Nova Scotia

Reprinted with permission.

Darce Changed the Conversation

Shortly after he began to write this column, we reached out to meet the man who was sharing his dementia journey. The stigma affiliated with a diagnosis of dementia is significant, and not everyone chooses to disclose their diagnosis so readily.

To learn of someone with Darce's insight and openness is a rare and beautiful thing. He normalized the range of emotions and symptoms he experienced and shared his strategies and reflections. We have countless conversations with clients that encourage self-compassion, but there's nothing quite like hearing it from a peer; especially one as eloquent and candid as Darce.

With great admiration, we referred to Darce as a "stigma buster"—his goal was to share his life living with dementia, and in doing so, inspire others to share and connect. Darce had more to offer than he needed in return. He helped us in many ways besides the column.

He served on our board for a short time, was a panelist at our early-stage forum and provincial conference (where he took the sails out of the interviewer by pre-empting their prepared questions the first chance he got to speak), presented to Dalhousie medical students, was the face of one of our fundraising campaigns, and was featured in a public service announcement to promote our Helpline. Darce not only changed the conversation, in many ways, he started the conversation in Nova Scotia. His legacy will help Nova Scotians impacted by dementia for years to come.

In his writing, Darce shares an incredible first-hand perspective. Early articles capture the early symptoms and behaviours that led to his diagnosis, promoting public awareness and recognition of warning signs. His journey also showcases the impact of accessing a timely diagnosis delivered with dignity, hope, and strategies.

One such strategy was the introduction of a fitness program and adoption of a cane to maintain his function and independence. Making physical activity a habit is a key step for people at any age or stage of life. Exercise can not only reduce one's risk of dementia, but also reduce the severity of symptoms post-diagnosis. Darce's honest account of his ups and downs humanizes the experience of adopting such behaviours in later life, particularly post-diagnosis.

Darce also adapted as his symptoms changed to maintain meaningful activities like urban walking and going to the local farmers' market. Many people with dementia describe withdrawing from society after a diagnosis due to encountering stigma as well as the challenges that dementia symptoms can bring. Darce made changes within his control, and called for broader system changes, too. His advocacy around the concept of dementia-friendliness influenced positive change for those with dementia and, more broadly, for all those living with disabilities in Nova Scotia.

Throughout his articles, we understand that Darce was well-supported by friends and family, and well-connected in his community. Dorothea and their children were a steady source of strength and motivation in maintaining "the essence of Darce."

For many who don't have such a natural support network in place after a diagnosis, the local Alzheimer Society is a helpful starting point in creating one. Doing so can provide timely access to information, education, and support from knowledgeable staff.

Dementia support lines provide confidential, individualized support and connection to a wide range of programs for people with dementia, their care partners, health care professionals, and the public.

The Alzheimer Society of Nova Scotia is the leading not-for-profit health charity serving Nova Scotians impacted by dementia. Active in communities across the province, the Society offers help for today through programs and services, and hope for tomorrow by funding research to find the cause and the cure. To find out more, visit alzheimer.ca/ns.

Emulating Darce

Darce Fardy made a major contribution to health care in Nova Scotia and beyond when he decided to invest a huge amount of time and energy over many years in informing the public of Nova Scotia on the challenges of having Alzheimer's.

His incredible ability and reputation as a journalist enabled him to communicate his experience with Alzheimer's in a way that enabled many thousands of people to understand that one can have an active and stimulating life after being diagnosed with Alzheimer's.

Historically, most people probably had the impression that such a diagnosis led to a life of not being worthwhile. Darce clearly demonstrated that, after diagnosis, he was able to be active, stimulating, and valued, adding to the lives of family, friends, and the general public of the province, as he did.

As a person who has recently been diagnosed with Alzheimer's, I hope to emulate his great example—informing Nova Scotians that life with Alzheimer's is not just worthwhile but positive and fun.

Robbie Shaw,
Alzheimer Society spokesperson living with dementia

Ten Ways to Reduce Your Risk of Dementia

On September 6, 2022, the Alzheimer Society of Canada released *Navigating the Path Forward for Dementia in Canada: The Landmark Study*—a new study forecasting dementia rates in Canada to 2050—including strategies on how we can take action now to improve our collective brain health.

Everybody has a role to play in this challenge of reducing future dementia rates, so this study lists actions for Alzheimer Societies, health systems, governments, researchers, and individuals to take. On the individual front, the Alzheimer Society recommends these ten evidence-based ways to reduce your risk of developing dementia.

1. **Be physically active each day.**
    Get moving! Walk, roll, jog, dance, swim, bike, garden, or do chores or yard work. Any physical activity is better than none at all.

2. **Protect, check, and support your hearing.**
    Hearing loss in midlife can increase dementia risk by an average of 90 percent. Use hearing aids if needed—they help reduce that risk. Protect your hearing from loud noises. Get your hearing tested.

3. **Stay socially active.**
    Stay connected and engaged with your family, friends, and community. Virtual visits and activities count, too! Social isolation in later life can increase dementia risk by an average of 60 percent.

4. **Manage your medical conditions and learn more about them.**
    In collaboration with your health care provider, try to manage complex conditions such as diabetes and obesity as best you can. These two conditions in particular can increase dementia risk, among others.

5. **Quit smoking.**
   Quitting or reducing smoking, even in later life, can improve your brain health and reduce your dementia risk. Ask your health care team for support!

6. **Seek support for depression.**
   Depression is more than just feeling sad. Seeking depression treatment and support will help improve your mood and brain functioning, as well as allowing you to take action on other risk factors.

7. **Drink less alcohol.**
   Research shows that drinking more than twelve standard drinks a week in midlife increases dementia risk by an average of 20 percent. Try out the growing number of mocktail and alcohol-free drink options instead! And if you need help with limiting alcohol, speak with your healthcare provider.

8. **Protect your heart.**
   Working with your health care provider, monitor and manage your blood pressure and heart health. What's good for the heart is also good for the brain!

9. **Avoid concussion and traumatic brain injury.**
   Steer clear of activities where you might put your brain at risk of harm. Follow traffic rules and pedestrian signals. Be aware of your surroundings. Play, travel, and work safe!

10. **Aim to get quality sleep.**
    Work toward sleeping well for six to eight hours each night. If you experience sleep apnea or other sleep issues, talk to your healthcare provider for treatment options.

Stigma Surrounding Dementia

Stigma prevents people living with dementia from living fully with dignity and respect. Help us fight stigma by learning more about its effects and taking steps to reduce its impact.

- Stigma against dementia encompasses any negative attitude or discriminatory behaviour against people living with dementia, solely on the basis of having the disease.
- When a disease is as prevalent as dementia, yet still poorly understood, it's easy for false beliefs to spread. Left unchallenged, these beliefs perpetuate stigmatizing attitudes against people living with dementia, reducing their quality of life.
- These attitudes extend to the families and caregivers of people living with dementia, affecting them as well.
- The unfortunate reality is that any person living with dementia is very likely to encounter stigma—even though dementia can affect anyone. No one is immune to the risks of dementia, and there is no cure or treatment that can guarantee prevention.
- People living with dementia did not choose to have this disease, and they certainly don't appreciate being labelled and ignored, among other negative responses, due to their diagnosis.

There are many ways that stigma can negatively impact the lives of people living with dementia, their families, and their caregivers:

- Lack of awareness about dementia
- Harmful and misleading assumptions
- Negative language
- Belittlement and jokes
- No support after diagnosis
- Stigma by association
- Loss of self-worth.

People living with dementia are experiencing stigma right now. Even though more than half a million Canadians live with dementia, many feel excluded, ignored, and treated differently for something beyond their control.

If you know a person living with dementia, chances are they've experienced discrimination that they wouldn't have faced if they didn't have dementia. Sadly, while most Canadians acknowledge that dementia is a serious disease, and that people living with dementia are likely to experience discrimination, attitudes that reinforce stigma against dementia are still common. There is perhaps no better way to know what stigma is than to listen to the people who have experienced it first-hand.

The Charter of Rights for People with Dementia

People living with dementia in Canada are entitled to the same human rights as any other person in Canada, as outlined in the Canadian Charter of Rights and Freedoms. However, stigma and discrimination are huge barriers for people with dementia and often contravene these rights.

That's why the Alzheimer Society supported the development of the first-ever Canadian Charter of Rights for People with Dementia. The landmark Charter is the culmination of over a year's work by the Alzheimer Society of Canada's Advisory Group of people with dementia, whose members represent different walks of life from across the country.

The Charter defines seven explicit rights to empower those living with dementia in Canada to self-advocate. It also ensures that the people and organizations will support and protect their rights.

Alzheimer *Society*

CANADIAN CHARTER OF RIGHTS FOR PEOPLE WITH DEMENTIA

As a person with dementia, I have the same human rights as every Canadian as outlined in the Canadian Charter of Rights and Freedoms. The following charter:

- Makes sure people with dementia know their rights,
- Empowers people with dementia to ensure their rights are protected and respected, and
- Makes sure that people and organizations that support people with dementia know these rights.

As a person with dementia, the following rights are especially important to me. I have the right:

1 To be free from discrimination of any kind.

2 To benefit from all of Canada's civic and legal rights.

3 To participate in developing and implementing policies that affect my life.

4 To access support so that I can live as independently as possible and be as engaged as possible in my community. This helps me:

- Meet my physical, cognitive, social, and spiritual needs,
- Get involved in community and civic opportunities, and
- Access opportunities for lifelong learning.

5 To get the information and support I need to participate as fully as possible in decisions that affect me, including care decisions from the point of diagnosis to palliative and end-of-life care.

6 To expect that professionals involved in my care are:

- Trained in both dementia and human rights.
- Held accountable for protecting my human rights including my right to get the support and information I need to make decisions that are right for me.
- Treating me with respect and dignity.
- Offering me equal access to appropriate treatment options as I develop health conditions other than my dementia.

7 To access effective complaint and appeal procedures when my rights are not protected or respected.

It will take the effort of every Canadian to protect and respect the rights of people with dementia so that we are seen as valuable and vital community members.

The Canadian Charter of Rights for People with Dementia (alzheimer.ca/charter). Courtesy Alzheimer Society of Canada Advisory Group.